Advances in
Brain Imaging

D1518620

Review of Psychiatry Series
John M. Oldham, M.D.
Michelle B. Riba, M.D., M.S.
Series Editors

Advances in Brain Imaging

EDITED BY

John M. Morihisa, M.D.

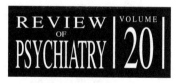

No. 4

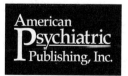

Washington, DC
London, England

Copyright © 2001 American Psychiatric Publishing, Inc.
04   03   02   01   4   3   2   1

ALL RIGHTS RESERVED
Manufactured in the United States of America on acid-free paper
First Edition

American Psychiatric Publishing, Inc.
1400 K Street, NW
Washington, DC 20005
www.appi.org

RC
473
.B7
A35
2001

The correct citation for this book is

Morihisa JM (editor): *Advances in Brain Imaging* (Review of Psychiatry Series, Volume 20, Number 4; Oldham JM and Riba MB, series editors). Washington, DC, American Psychiatric Publishing, 2001

Library of Congress Cataloging-in-Publication Data
Advances in brain imaging / edited by John M. Morihisa.
    p. ; cm. — (Review of psychiatry ; v. 20, no. 4)
    Includes bibliographical references and index.
    ISBN 1-58562-028-9 (alk. paper)
    1. Brain—Imaging. 2. Mental illness—Diagnosis. I. Morihisa, John M., 1951–
II. Review of psychiatry series ; v. 20, 4.
    [DNLM: 1. Mental Disorders—diagnosis. 2. Brain—physiopathology. 3. Brain Mapping—methods. 4. Diagnostic Imaging—methods. 5. Psychiatry—methods. WM 141
A2445 2001]
    RC473.B7 A35 2001
    616.89'075—dc21
                                                                        2001016043

British Library Cataloguing in Publication Data
A CIP record is available from the British Library.

Cover photograph: Copyright © 2001 Custom Medical Stock Photo, Inc.

Contents

Contributors   ix

Introduction to the Review of Psychiatry Series   xi
John M. Oldham, M.D., and
Michelle B. Riba, M.D., M.S., Series Editors

Foreword   xv
John M. Morihisa, M.D.

Chapter 1
Functional Brain Imaging in
Psychiatry: The Next Wave   1
Joseph H. Callicott, M.D.
    Functional Magnetic Resonance
      Imaging (fMRI) in Psychiatry   3
    A Dynamic Approach to Brain
      Mapping in Psychiatry   8
    Magnetic Resonance and Genetic Susceptibility   15
    Conclusions   17
    References   18

Chapter 2
Cognitive Neuroscience: The New
Neuroscience of the Mind and
Its Implications for Psychiatry   25
Cameron S. Carter, M.D.
    Executive Functions and the Brain   27
    ACC and Performance Monitoring   29
    DLPFC and Top-Down Control   32
    Impaired Executive Functions in
      Schizophrenia: Role of DLPFC and ACC   36
    DLPFC and Impaired Executive
      Functions in Schizophrenia   38

ACC and Impaired Performance
Monitoring in Schizophrenia 41
Overcontrol and Dysfunctional Performance
Monitoring in OCD: Role of the ACC 43
Conclusions 45
References 47

Chapter 3
**Functional Magnetic Resonance Imaging in
Children and Adolescents: Implications for
Research on Emotion** 53
Daniel S. Pine, M.D.
Developmental Psychopathology Perspectives
Applied to Mood and Anxiety Disorders 55
Data Implicating Neural Circuits in
Pediatric Mood and Anxiety Disorders 59
Using fMRI to Probe Developmental
Dysfunction in Neural Circuits 66
Conclusions 74
References 75

Chapter 4
**Brain Structure and Function in
Late-Life Depression** 83
Harold A. Sackeim, Ph.D.
Brain Structural Abnormalities: Encephalomalacia 84
Etiology of Encephalomalacia 91
Pathophysiology of Encephalomalacia 94
Volumetric Brain Structural Abnormalities 97
Functional Brain Abnormalities 105
Treatment and Recovery Effects in
Late-Life Depression 110
Conclusions 113
References 115

Chapter 5
Neuroimaging Studies of Major Depression   **123**
  Wayne C. Drevets, M.D.
    Overview of the Imaging Research Program   124
    Neurophysiological Imaging
      Studies of Major Depression   127
    Functional Anatomical Correlates of Depression   138
    Anatomic Circuits Implicated in MDD   153
    Histopathological Findings in the
      L-T-C and L-C-S-P-T Circuits   154
    Clinical Implications and
      Directions for Future Studies   158
    References   159

Afterword   **171**
  John M. Morihisa, M.D.

Index   **175**

Contributors

Joseph H. Callicott, M.D.
Chief, Unit on Functional MRI, Clinical Brain Disorders Branch, National Institute of Mental Health/National Institutes of Health, Bethesda, Maryland

Cameron S. Carter, M.D.
Associate Professor, Department of Psychiatry, University of Pittsburgh, Pittsburgh, Pennsylvania

Wayne C. Drevets, M.D.
Chief, Mood and Anxiety Disorders Section, NIMH, Bethesda, Maryland; Associate Professor, Departments of Psychiatry and Radiology, University of Pittsburgh, Pittsburgh, Pennsylvania

John M. Morihisa, M.D.
Professor, Department of Psychiatry, Albany Medical College; Capital District Psychiatric Center, Albany, New York

John M. Oldham, M.D.
Dollard Professor and Acting Chairman, Department of Psychiatry, Columbia University College of Physicians and Surgeons, New York, New York

Daniel S. Pine, M.D.
Head of Developmental Studies, Program on Mood and Anxiety, Intramural Research Program, National Institute of Mental Health, Bethesda, Maryland

Michelle B. Riba, M.D., M.S.
Associate Chair for Education and Academic Affairs, Department of Psychiatry, University of Michigan Medical School, Ann Arbor, Michigan

Harold A. Sackeim, Ph.D.
Chief, Department of Biological Psychiatry, New York State Psychiatric Institute; Professor, Departments of Psychiatry and Radiology, College of Physicians and Surgeons of Columbia University, New York

Introduction to the Review of Psychiatry Series

John M. Oldham, M.D., and
Michelle B. Riba, M.D., M.S., Series Editors

2001 REVIEW OF PSYCHIATRY SERIES TITLES

- *PTSD in Children and Adolescents*
  EDITED BY SPENCER ETH, M.D.
- *Integrated Treatment of Psychiatric Disorders*
  EDITED BY JERALD KAY, M.D.
- *Somatoform and Factitious Disorders*
  EDITED BY KATHARINE A. PHILLIPS, M.D.
- *Treatment of Recurrent Depression*
  EDITED BY JOHN F. GREDEN, M.D.
- *Advances in Brain Imaging*
  EDITED BY JOHN M. MORIHISA, M.D.

In today's rapidly changing world, the dissemination of information is one of its rapidly changing elements. Information virtually assaults us, and proclaimed experts abound. Witness, for example, the 2000 presidential election in the United States, during which instant opinions were plentiful about the previously obscure science of voting machines, the electoral college, and the meaning of the words of the highest court in the land. For medicine the situation is the same: the World Wide Web virtually bulges with health advice, treatment recommendations, and strident warnings about the dangers of this approach or that. Authoritative and reliable guides to help the consumer differentiate between sound advice and unsubstantiated opinion are hard to come by, and our patients and their families may be misled by bad information without even knowing it.

At no time has it been more important, then, for psychiatrists and other clinicians to be well informed, armed with the very latest findings, and well versed in evidence-based medicine. We have designed Volume 20 of the Review of Psychiatry Series with these trends in mind—to be, if you will, a how-to manual: how to accurately identify illnesses, how to understand where they come from and what is going wrong in specific conditions, how to measure the extent of the problem, and how to design the best treatment, especially for the particularly difficult-to-treat disorders.

The central importance of stress as a pathogen in major mental illness throughout the life cycle is increasingly clear. One form of stress is *trauma*. Extreme trauma can lead to illness at any age, but its potential to set the stage badly for life when severe trauma occurs during early childhood is increasingly recognized. In *PTSD in Children and Adolescents*, Spencer Eth and colleagues review the evidence from animal and human studies of the aberrations, both psychological and biological, that can persist throughout adulthood as a result of trauma experienced during childhood. Newer technologies have led to new knowledge of the profound nature of some of these changes, from persistently altered stress hormones to gene expression and altered protein formation. In turn, hypersensitivities result from this early stress-induced biological programming, so that cognitive and emotional symptom patterns emerge rapidly in reaction to specific environmental stimuli.

Nowhere in the field of medicine is technology advancing more rapidly than in brain imaging, generating a level of excitement that surely surpasses the historical moment when the discovery of the X ray first allowed us to noninvasively see into the living human body. The new imaging methods, fortunately, do not involve the risk of radiation exposure, and the capacity of the newest imaging machines to reveal brain structure and function in great detail is remarkable. Yet in many ways these techniques still elude clinical application, since they are expensive and increasingly complex to administer and interpret. John Morihisa has gathered a group of our best experts to discuss the latest developments in *Advances in Brain Imaging*, and the shift toward greater clinical utility is clear in their descriptions of these methods. Perhaps most intriguing is the promise that through these methods we can identify, before the onset of symptoms, those most at risk of developing psychiatric disorders, as discussed by Daniel Pine regarding childhood disorders and by Harold Sackeim regarding late-life depression.

Certain conditions, such as the somatoform and factitious disorders, can baffle even our most experienced clinicians. As Katharine Phillips points out in her foreword to *Somatoform and Factitious Disorders*, these disorders frequently go unrecognized or are misdiagnosed, and patients with these conditions may be seen more often in the offices of nonpsychiatric physicians than in those of psychiatrists. Although these conditions have been reported throughout the recorded history of medicine, patients with these disorders either are fully convinced that their problems are "physical" instead of "mental" or choose to present their problems that way. In this book, experienced clinicians provide guidelines to help identify the presence of the somatoform and factitious disorders, as well as recommendations about their treatment.

Treatment of all psychiatric disorders is always evolving, based on new findings and clinical experience; at times, the field has become polarized, with advocates of one approach vying with advocates of another (e.g., psychotherapy versus pharmacotherapy). Patients, however, have the right to receive the best treatment available, and most of the time the best treatment includes psychotherapy *and* pharmacotherapy, as detailed in *Integrated Treatment of Psychiatric Disorders*. Jerald Kay and colleagues propose the term *integrated treatment* for this approach, a recommended fundamental of treatment planning. Psychotherapy alone, of course, may be the best treatment for some patients, just as pharmacotherapy may be the mainstay of treatment for others, but in all cases there should be thoughtful consideration of a combination of these approaches.

Finally, despite tremendous progress in the treatment of most psychiatric disorders, there are some conditions that are stubbornly persistent in spite of the best efforts of our experts. John Greden takes up one such area in *Treatment of Recurrent Depres-*

sion, referring to recurrent depression as one of the most disabling disorders of all, so that, in his opinion, "a call to arms" is needed. Experienced clinicians and researchers review optimal treatment approaches for this clinical population. As well, new strategies, such as vagus nerve stimulation and minimally invasive brain stimulation, are reviewed, indicating the need to go beyond our currently available treatments for these seriously ill patients.

All in all, we believe that Volume 20 admirably succeeds in advising us how to do the best job that can be done at this point to diagnose, understand, measure, and treat some of the most challenging conditions that prompt patients to seek psychiatric help.

Foreword

John M. Morihisa, M.D.

In this new century the field of brain imaging will evolve and grow to fulfill the bright promise it has showed from its beginning over a generation ago. This book includes the work of five scientists who are contributing to that growth by investigating a spectrum of psychopathologies using a variety of imaging approaches. All have brought to the scientific process a mastery of the technological issues melded with an abiding interest in the underlying theory. As a result, their research and writing have the utility and clarity that are crucial to the explication of the highly complex issues at the foundations of brain imaging.

These writers discuss psychopathologies ranging from major depression and obsessive-compulsive disorder to schizophrenia. In so doing they report some of the most recent findings in the field, review the relevant data in the literature, and place this research in a critical neuroscience context, demonstrating how basic neuroscience research has shaped their application of brain imaging to questions in psychiatry.

Although quite disparate clinical disorders are discussed, there are convergences in the neuropathological substrates highlighted. These convergences may help delineate useful disease pathways based upon pathophysiological correlates that may complement nosology. If successful, this work will build neural-network models of the ways in which the brain malfunctions for each disease. From these models enhanced therapeutic tools might be developed.

These scientists also examine a broad range of patient populations, from the pediatric to the geriatric. This diversity of investigations enables us to begin to see patterns woven through different technical approaches and various psychopathologies.

As a result, certain neural circuits, such as those in areas of the prefrontal lobes, are further characterized as to their potential role in the pathophysiology of mental illness.

What is gained in the end is an enhanced understanding of the theory and practice of brain imaging in psychiatry and an exciting glimpse of the future of both the technology and the science. This future will include not only new technology but also novel applications of existing technology. One example of a different approach is Drevets's compelling longitudinal and multidisciplinary investigation of major depression (see Chapter 5).

In Chapter 1, Callicott provides an excellent discussion of functional magnetic resonance imaging (fMRI), including a valuable review of its strengths and limitations. He shares with us some of the difficulties of the earlier generation of brain-imaging findings and points out that most were a challenge to interpret due to their lack of clinical or neuropathological correlations. Further, he emphasizes the importance of applying the perspective of a continuum of performance levels when devising research paradigms employing cognitive activation. Callicott describes the combined use of fMRI and proton magnetic resonance spectroscopic imaging, a "presumptive measure of neuronal pathology," to provide additional confidence that abnormal brain images actually correlate with brain pathology. In addition to emphasizing the therapeutic implications of brain-imaging findings, Callicott also suggests that this field may achieve its greatest utility in the search for the genetic bases of psychiatric disorders. Indeed, Callicott's most exciting theme is the future application of brain imaging in concert with genetic findings. He gives useful examples of this approach; for example, studies of schizophrenia that employ abnormalities of neurophysiology to establish genetic linkage. He concludes that the search for specific neuropathology, rather than pathognomic findings, may be the most fruitful application of brain imaging.

In Chapter 2, Carter emphasizes the importance of cognitive deficits to our understanding of psychiatric disorders. Indeed, he points out that deficits in cognition can be powerful predictors of the degree of return-to-function in some psychiatric illnesses. Carter goes on to describe fascinating developments in cognitive neuroscience that are important to the field of brain imaging. Neuroimaging researchers have been able to build upon the basic work of cognitive neuroscience to assist in the interpretation of functional brain imaging findings. Carter then emphasizes that when taken together, the work in these two fields of science raise the hope of more efficacious therapeutic approaches to the cognitive disabilities of our patients. Employing the conceptual context of impaired executive function, Carter uses neuroscience findings to examine and interpret neuroimaging data from studies of schizophrenia and obsessive-compulsive disorder. From these data he develops an exciting theory of altered executive function, which may be at the heart of both of these challenging psychiatric illnesses. This work may lead not only to a better understanding of these disorders but also to the development of new therapeutic approaches for them, if we can delineate elements of the pathophysiology of each illness.

Pine, in Chapter 3, tells of a compelling new way to investigate disorders of emotion in children that utilizes a synthesis of neuroscience, psychiatry, and developmental psychology. He feels that fMRI may be uniquely powerful in the delineation of the underlying pathophysiology of psychiatric disorders in the pediatric population such as major depression, generalized anxiety disorder, separation anxiety disorder, and social phobia. Pine poses intriguing research questions concerning the application of brain-imaging technology to the study of children. In this way he builds a compelling argument for exploring the utility of placing anxiety and mood disorders in the conceptual context of human development when devising investigational paradigms. Moreover, he feels that fMRI may help us to determine the variables that characterize children at risk for mood and anxiety disorders as adults. Finally, Pine believes that basic neuroscience research on the neural substrates of emotion can suggest new approaches to the investigation of anxiety and mood disorders and thereby fundamentally altering the way we conceptualize these illnesses.

In Chapter 4, Sackeim presents both structural and functional brain imaging findings in patients with late-life depression. He reports that there is growing evidence suggesting that patients with this disorder demonstrate an excess of hyperintensities on magnetic resonance imaging (MRI). Further, Sackeim discusses findings of decreased brain volume and of abnormalities of regional cerebral blood flow in late-life depression and examines how they compare to those of younger patients with major depression. He also raises an intriguing question of trait-versus-state in some of the abnormalities seen in late-life depression. Sackeim suggests that these findings may lead to important insights in diagnosis, treatment response, and prognosis for late-life depression.

Finally, Drevets describes an investigation of major depression that uses a strikingly multidisciplinary approach allying positron emission tomography and MRI with complementary neuroscience approaches such as histopathology to provide a panoply of correlative data. He and his colleagues have documented abnormalities of glucose metabolism and cerebral blood flow in a number of brain regions, including the prefrontal cortex. Of special interest is his description of the changes in these abnormalities after therapeutic intervention. Drevets is able to delineate some abnormalities in depression that appear to depend upon the mood of the patient and other neurophysiologic differences that persist even after treatment. Each category of these findings has interesting possibilities for our understanding of the underlying pathophysiology of depression. Moreover, Drevets offers an especially comprehensive and detailed review of the literature and places this work in its appropriate neurobiological context. Perhaps one of the most distinctive characteristics of this particular chapter is the strength of its research design, which demonstrates a longitudinal and intensely multimodal neuroscience approach that is particularly well-suited to studies of the brain.

Each of these chapters tells a fascinating story of new concepts and approaches, stirring our anticipation of future scientific advances. When taken together, moreover, they begin to inspire one of the most valuable emotions that can be felt by researchers or clinicians in our field: hope for advancement in therapeutic interventions for our patients.

Chapter 1

Functional Brain Imaging in Psychiatry

The Next Wave

Joseph H. Callicott, M.D.

Early failure to identify brain lesions in psychiatric disorders led to the conceptualization of these diseases as *functional* as opposed to classic *organic* conditions like stroke. Recent research has removed this erroneous dichotomization, but the ascendancy of the neurological or organic-lesion model has been a mixed blessing. Certainly, neuropathological deficits will be found for most psychiatric disorders; however, they will likely be subtle, involving alterations of cellular function, communication, or connectivity rather than pronounced tissue loss. For example, Selemon et al. (1998) reported significant but small neuropathological changes in the postmortem schizophrenic brain, with cortical thinning of approximately 8% and an approximately 21% increase in neuronal density (decrease in neuropil).

The original intent of in vivo functional brain imaging was to illuminate the underlying physiological disturbances that lead to manifest illness. Based on the neurological tradition, alterations in cerebral blood flow or metabolic rate were presumed to mark the brain lesions underlying loss of function. However, no independent measures were available to justify this presumption of a one-to-one correlation between abnormal imaging data and underlying neuronal pathology. Furthermore, these functional imaging abnormalities have not proven disorder specific enough to allow reliable functional-pathological correlations. Without such correlations, the application of functional imaging to psychiatric clinical practice will be difficult.

The history of reduced prefrontal cortex (PFC) function in schizophrenia is an illustrative example of this conundrum. Initially identified in patients at rest by Ingvar and Franzen (1974), reduced PFC function has been most reliably identified in schizophrenic patients studied while performing PFC-dependent cognitive tasks such as the Wisconsin Card Sorting Test (Weinberger and Berman 1996). In combination with neuropathological and structural imaging data suggesting PFC pathology, these data seemed a reasonable candidate for a pathognomonic marker of underlying prefrontal pathology. However, whereas schizophrenic patients generally perform poorly on such prefrontal tasks, there are reports of normal (Curtis et al. 1999; Frith et al. 1995; Mellers et al. 1998), decreased (Callicott et al. 1998b; Carter et al. 1998; Curtis et al. 1998; Fletcher et al. 1998; Franzen and Ingvar 1975; Stevens et al. 1998; Weinberger et al. 1988, 1992; Yurgelun-Todd et al. 1996), and increased prefrontal blood flow in schizophrenia (Callicott et al. 2000b; Manoach et al. 1999, 2000; Stevens et al. 1998). Ragland et al. (1998) reported both reduced and intact PFC regional cerebral blood flow in a cohort of schizophrenic patients given two different prefrontal tasks: an executive memory task (i.e., Wisconsin Card Sorting Test) and a declarative memory task (i.e., Paired Associate Recognition Test). In a similar vein, Bullmore et al. (1999) reported both attenuated and normal PFC activation in a group of schizophrenic patients during a single scanning session, with patients being given both a covert semantic decision task (normal PFC activation) and a covert verbal fluency task (attenuated PFC activation).

Certainly, experimental variables such as choice of cognitive task, small sample size, and variability in antipsychotic medication status could be invoked to explain such discrepancies. However, a final blow to the presumption that reduced prefrontal blood-flow findings reflect PFC pathology came with the recent demonstration that reduced prefrontal function is a correlate of reduced performance in healthy comparison subjects. Using a dual task paradigm, Goldberg et al. (1998) found that prefrontal blood flow and performance decreased as healthy subjects simultaneously performed the Wisconsin Card Sorting Test and an auditory shadowing task. In a more direct exploration of varying performance, Callicott et al. (1999) explored the prefrontal response to increasing WM (working memory) load that eventually exceeded the WM capacity of healthy subjects. They found evidence for an inverted U-shaped curve of PFC activation that began to slope downward over the range of WM difficulty exceeding healthy WM capacity. Reduced PFC activity coincident with reduced behavioral capacity has been found in single-unit recording studies in nonhuman primates during WM tasks (Funahashi et al. 1989, 1991) and in electrophysiological studies in humans attempting complex motor tasks (Gevins et al. 1987). A further illustration is a study by Fletcher et al. (1998) in which they found hypofrontality only when a parametrically increasing word list recall task went beyond the patients' memory capacity.

Given the growing evidence for PFC pathology in schizophrenia, it would be unwise to simply abandon functional brain mapping due to such inconsistencies. Rather, we will examine an alternative approach to mapping the effects of presumptive neuropathology in psychiatric illnesses like schizophrenia. In addition, we will examine the use of proton magnetic resonance spectroscopic imaging (^{1}H-MRSI) as a method for connecting functional findings with neuronal pathology. Finally, in contrast to previous attempts to construe functional imaging findings as diagnostically relevant, we will discuss the use of such findings to guide the search for the genetic underpinnings of neuropsychiatric illness.

Functional Magnetic Resonance Imaging (fMRI) in Psychiatry

Advantages such as minimal invasiveness, no radioactivity, widespread availability, and virtually unlimited study repetitions make fMRI ideally suited to the study of in vivo brain function in psychiatry (Levin et al. 1995). Before proceeding to the findings themselves, however, it is important to be mindful of the continued limitations of fMRI brain mapping (Weinberger et al. 1996). Due to the simple fact that psychiatric patients move during fMRI exams, psychiatric fMRI investigations require increased vigilance for potential artifacts. Because fMRI results are presented as statistical maps, failure to systematically control for artifact will remain invisible to the reader and render any such work difficult to interpret. Put simply, patient motion during scanning is deleterious based on the small contrast-to-noise ratio present in most fMRI studies, with signal magnitude typically ranging from 3%–5% on 1.5 T clinical MRI magnets. Motion introduces increased variance, which unpredictably increases or decreases apparent activation on statistical fMRI maps. In addition, excess motion (and occasional artifacts due to technical failure of the scanner) is not correctable using traditional solutions for interscan motion in fMRI (e.g., registration of images). Ultimately, the only solution is to exclude those studies with excessive artifact—although such artifact is often detected only after lengthy data processing and thus is not always amendable by repeat scanning.

For example, we studied a group of 10 matched schizophrenic patients and control subjects using the N-back working memory test (Callicott et al. 1998b). N-back working memory tasks typically present subjects with strings of letters or numbers that are encoded and then recalled; for example, on a 2-back task subjects recall stimuli seen two steps earlier in the sequence. Following the usual analysis steps (including image registration with no apparent interscan motion), we noted the predicted reduced prefrontal activation in patients. However, based on an earlier, failed study with schizophrenic patients where data were contaminated by movement, we modified the typical N-back protocol by requiring subjects to make a continual motor response throughout the study. We reasoned that if this "quality control" signal in contralateral sensorimotor cortex were absent (in spite of evidence that subjects were making responses) then there were likely "hidden" artifacts within the data requiring the exclusion of these subjects. When we found an apparent reduction in sensorimotor cortex activation in schizophrenic patients in spite of an equal number of motor responses between groups, we examined our data more closely. We found that although we had removed residual subject motion using registration, this process could not remove systematic group differences in signal intensity variance. We then created histogram plots of variance in fMRI signal throughout the brain during the experiment for each subject and excluded those subjects with increased variance. After matching for variance, we found identical motor cortex activation between groups. This allowed us to conclude that reduced prefrontal activation in the remaining schizophrenic patients was a result of PFC pathology and not simply an experimental artifact.

Another approach to this problem has been developed by Bullmore et al. (1999) and utilizes the fact that data are acquired in a periodic (on-off) design. When calculating fundamental power-quotient maps that identify signal that varies at the fundamental frequency of the periodic task design, Bullmore and colleagues identified any subject movement that also occurred in sync with the on-off design (so-called *stimulus-correlated motion* or SCM), such as motion introduced by motor responses or by visual tracking of stimuli. SCM can be compared across groups or controlled for in the statistical analysis. One limitation of this method, however, is that motion occurs in both a periodic and aperiodic fashion so that SCM may miss large infrequent motions that might still interfere with overall variance. Another alternative would be to use derived measures of artifact (e.g., amount of motion) as a covariate in statistical analyses such as statistical parametric mapping or multiple regression. A note of caution is in order, however, since our experience would suggest that beyond certain limits, artifact will increase variance to a level that renders statistical comparisons meaningless.

Perhaps as a result of historical precedent, the majority of fMRI studies of mental illness have been done on schizophrenia. The earliest fMRI explorations of schizophrenia tended to involve simple stimulus paradigms (e.g., photic stimulation) and repetitive motor movement (e.g., finger tapping). With photic stimulation, patients with schizophrenia were noted to have an exaggerated activation response within primary visual cortex (Renshaw et al. 1994). Similarly, Cohen et al. (1995), using dynamic susceptibility contrast MRI, found significantly increased regional cerebral blood volume in the left occipital cortex and left caudate of schizophrenic subjects. Possible interpretations include fundamental anomalies in cerebral vasculature in schizophrenia, alteration in the relationship between evoked neuronal activity and blood flow response as a consequence of schizophrenia or medications, alterations in apparent blood flow or volume due to alterations in the ratio of gray to white matter (partial volume effects), or an artifact of experimental design (e.g., patients blinking less because of medication effects). Using labeled-water positron emission tomography (^{15}O-H$_2$O PET), Taylor et al. (1997) were unable to replicate either increased blood volume or increased magnitude of response to photic stimulation of schizophrenic patients. However, they did find a greater spatial extent of activation. In the end, these abnormalities, if real, are difficult to interpret given the lack of compelling clinical or neuropathological data to support a priori assumptions of underlying pathology of the occipital cortex. Arnold et al. (1995) and Rajkowska et al. (1998) failed to find evidence of gross neuropathology, although Selemon et al. (1995) did report a 10% decrease in neuronal density in Brodmann area 17 in patients with schizophrenia.

Motor abnormalities in schizophrenia are perhaps easier to interpret based on evidence for minor neurological anomalies in schizophrenia. Two studies have found decreased magnitude of fMRI activation and a less lateralized response (Schroder et al. 1995; Wenz et al. 1994). Schroder et al. (1999) have replicated the finding of reduced activation. Mattay et al. (1997) also reported reduced laterality using complex self-guided motor movements but did not find a reduction in magnitude within the contralateral motor cortex. A major limitation of these studies was the use of antipsychotic medication, for which movement abnormalities are a major side effect. Thus, two follow-up studies failed to find differences in lateralization or magnitude of activation in unmedicated subjects (Braus et al. 1999, 2000). In fact, Buckley et al. (1997) failed to find evidence for reduced motor cortex activation in medicated patients, although lateralization was not presented. In two unmedicated catatonic schizophrenic patients, Northoff et al. (1999) found reduced activation, although subjects were given a benzodiazepine immediately prior to scanning. The ultimate import of these findings, if the effects they report are not due to medication, is unclear. Neuropathological examination of postmortem motor cortex has revealed both abnormal and normal cortex (Benes et al. 1986; Bogerts et al. 1993).

Several studies have investigated the impact of positive symptoms, specifically auditory hallucinations, on cortical function. David et al. (1996) and Woodruff et al. (1997) found abnormal temporal cortex activation in response to external speech in patients with schizophrenia. In two schizophrenic patients with auditory hallucinations, David et al. found reduced activation within auditory cortex in response to auditory stimuli but no abnormalities in visual cortex in response to visual stimuli. Woodruff et al. replicated this reduction of auditory cortex response in a larger sample of patients with auditory hallucinations. They interpreted their findings as meaning that the auditory hallucinations "competed" with the auditory stimuli for the cortical physiological response. In perhaps the most intriguing attempt to date to localize auditory hallucinations, Dierks et al. (1999) studied three hallucinating patients using a modified event-related design. Patients indicated when they were hallucinating, and fMRI data from these temporal epochs were analyzed. Dierks and colleagues identified an area within the primary auditory cortex (Heschl's gyrus) that was also activated by external auditory stimuli, suggesting that such hallucinations involve primary auditory cortex dysfunction.

Most studies in schizophrenia have been directed at prefrontal cortical dysfunction. The first report was by Yurgelun-Todd et al. (1996), who identified left prefrontal underactivation during word generation. Although limited by the use of a surface coil, this study has been replicated by Curtis et al. (1998). Volz et al. (1999) also demonstrated reduced PFC activation during the Continuous Performance Test. Callicott et al. (1998a) have reported decreased PFC activation in patients with impoverished WM, but increased activation in patients with relatively intact WM (Callicott et al. 2000b). In the latter report, other areas evincing an abnormal response included the anterior cingulate cortex and parietal cortex. Using the Sternberg Item Recognition Paradigm, Manoach et al. (1999, 2000) have twice reported increased PFC activation in the face of diminished recall accuracy. In the latter study, schizophrenic patients were found to activate basal ganglia and thalamus, in contradistinction to control subjects. In addition to reduced PFC activity during word generation (noted above), Curtis et al. (1999) found no difference in PFC activity during a semantic decision task. Stevens et al. (1998) found reduced ventral PFC activation during a verbal WM task. On balance, these diverse findings argue for dysfunction of PFC in schizophrenia, but the particular flavor (over- or underactivation) depends heavily on the nature and demands of a given task.

There have been a number of clever investigations of the limbic system. In a seminal study, Breiter et al. (1996) demonstrated increased limbic system activation (i.e., in the amygdala and orbitofrontal and cingulate cortices) with obsessive-compulsive disorder by exposing subjects to stimuli specific to their individual obsessions or compulsions while the subjects were in the scanner. Functional MRI has also been used to map locations within the limbic system that are stimulated by intoxication (e.g., nucleus accumbens, striatum, and prefrontal cortex; Breiter et al. 1997) or craving (e.g., prefrontal and cingulate cortices; Maas et al. 1998). Schneider et al. (1998) found reduced activation of the amygdala in schizophrenic patients during sad-mood induction. In a similar vein, Phillips et al. (1999) identified a number of activation differences between control subjects and schizophrenic patients within the limbic system (including the amygdala) in response to exposure to neutral, angry, and fearful faces.

A Dynamic Approach to Brain Mapping in Psychiatry

One explanation of the inconsistencies in the functional imaging literature rests in the observation that these studies have tended to examine brain function at a fixed level of difficulty, usually at maximum accuracy in given cognitive tasks. The study of the human brain at rest using blood flow techniques has largely been abandoned due to criticisms that "rest" is a complex mental state in its own right (Weinberger and Berman 1996). However, cognitive function and cognitive deficits exist along a continuum; even the most severely ill patient is capable of mustering some prefrontal cortical function. Thus, an alternative interpretation of the mélange of findings is that all may be valid reflections of different parts of the same continuum. For example, patients and control subjects may evince similar brain activation at low difficulty. As difficulty (or mental effort) increase, there appears to be a point at which performance differs somewhat, but patients activate to a greater extent than control subjects as a reflection of greater mental effort or of inefficient use of cortical resources. At a point where performance differences are marked, patient activation may be much less than that of healthy control subjects, who are able to muster greater cortical resources in service of the task. Finally, as the task surpasses healthy capacity, activation in control subjects will also drop (Callicott et al. 1999). The key to appreciating the impact of prefrontal cortical pathology on activation would then lie in an overall grasp of this dynamic continuum, rather than in simple comparisons of greater or lesser activation at any one part of the difficulty curve. The clinical analogy would be the use of graded exercise stress tests in the diagnosis of cardiac disease. In such tests, cardiologists do not simply use a measure of maximal effort. Maximal effort achieved and the physiological response to increasing effort *together* characterize cardiac function, thus guiding the use of medications, surgical intervention, or both. Like brain-imaging paradigms, cardiac stress tests are not diagnostic per se (e.g., do not differentiate two-vessel from three-vessel coronary artery disease or from the effects of a congenital myopathy). In the same way, we might conceive of our prefrontal cognitive tasks as mental treadmills by which we gauge prefrontal function. With its increased flexibility, fMRI may allow us to map a sufficiently wide dynamic range. Having done so, we might be able to gauge the relative importance of associated issues, such as medication usage, that are also difficult to gauge using only one point from this hypothetical prefrontal function curve.

An additional benefit of the dynamic mapping approach is that it may generate findings in illnesses in which neural pathology does not produce deficits as pronounced as those of schizophrenia. A recent study of the impact of genetic variability and cognitive dysfunction illustrates this point. M.F. Egan et al. (unpublished observations, 2000) examined the relationship of prefrontal function in patients with schizophrenia, in their unaffected siblings, and in healthy control subjects to catechol O-methyltransferase (COMT) genotype. A single nucleotide variant in COMT (Val108→Met158) confers a fourfold increase in enzymatic activity over the ancestral form (Val-Val). The variant enzyme also clears dopamine at a much faster rate than the heterozygous (Val-Met) or homozygous (Met-Met) forms (Mannisto and Kaakkola 1999). Of all groups, Met-Met individuals performed the best on the Wisconsin Card Sorting Test. Functional MRI data taken from control subjects and schizophrenic patients showed a dramatic increase in prefrontal efficiency (reduced activation) during the N-back WM task for Met-Met individuals, with heterozygous Val-Met individuals intermediate between Met-Met and Val-Val individuals (despite equal task performance across genotypes). Whereas performance on the WM task alone would have missed the functional consequences of COMT genotype, fMRI was able to distinguish this subtle physiological effect. The same may be true for the milder cognitive deficits associated with bipolar disorder or major depressive disorder. Functional MRI might be sensitive to the functional consequences of these disorders, where neuropsychological testing alone might miss such pathophysiology.

Ultimately, the value of more subtle functional differences will rest with evidence that a given cortical or subcortical region is a likely candidate for pathology. Cortical stress tests sensitive to the function of a candidate region can then be selected and used for screening. Schizophrenia again offers an illustrative example. There is little debate that PFC neuronal pathology exists in schizophrenia and that this pathology may be more prominent in dorsal PFC (Brodmann areas 9 and 46). Suspicions of PFC dysfunction date back to clinical observations noting the similarities between the negative or deficit symptoms in schizophrenic patients and those of patients with frontal lobe lesions (Kraepelin 1919; Piercy 1964). Postmortem neuropathology has found PFC abnormalities such as reduced neuropil (intraneuronal volume) without neuronal loss in dorsal PFC (Brodmann areas 9 and 46; Selemon et al. 1995; Selemon et al. 1998), reductions in the abundance and metabolic activity of dorsal PFC interneurons (Akbarian et al. 1996; Benes et al. 1991), and diminished inhibitory inputs from prefrontal chandelier cells onto the axonal processes of dorsal PFC pyramidal neurons (Woo et al. 1998). In vivo ^{1}H-MRSI studies have repeatedly found reduced concentrations of the intraneuronal chemical N-acetylaspartate (NAA) in dorsal PFC (Bertolino et al. 1996, 1998a, 1998b; Cecil et al. 1999; Thomas et al. 1998). Finally, decreased NAA (decreased neuronal integrity) in dorsal PFC is predictive of negative symptoms in schizophrenia ($r > -0.50$; Callicott et al. 2000a). Neurophysiological experiments in schizophrenic patients and those with brain lesions have noted abnormal eye-tracking function referable to dorsal PFC (Holzman et al. 1973) and altered PFC electroencephalographic patterns (Abrams and Taylor 1979), including a disruption of normal coherence between PFC and other brain regions (Tauscher et al. 1998). Thus, there exists ample a priori evidence to direct attention to PFC function. Prior to examining our dynamic approach to brain mapping, however, it is important to understand the contribution ^{1}H-MRSI data have made to the assessment of fMRI findings.

^{1}H-MRSI now offers the ability to directly correlate abnormal imaging findings with a presumptive measure of neuronal pathology as an a posteriori confirmation that abnormal findings imply abnormal neurons. ^{1}H-MRSI is a whole-brain proton magnetic resonance spectroscopy (^{1}H-MRS) technique (Bertolino et al. 1996) that acquires four 15-mm slabs of brain with a nominal resolution at 1.5 T of approximately 7.5 mm x 7.5 mm x 15 mm. Like structural imaging, ^{1}H-MRS relies on regional differences in proton (^{1}H) concentration. Whereas structural MRI relies on mainly tissue water, which represents the largest peak on a spectrum of tissue protons, ^{1}H-MRS looks for quantitative differences in protons attached to various abundant chemical moieties that exist as smaller peaks in the proton spectrum once the large water signal is suppressed (most commonly NAA; choline-containing compounds, and creatine + phosphocreatine). Fortuitously, NAA is a neuron-specific surrogate marker of cellular integrity (Tsai and Coyle 1995) whose relative abundance is likely linked to mitochondrial metabolism (Jenkins et al. 2000). NAA levels have been examined in numerous neurological disorders where relative increases and decreases readily track illness progression and treatment (Tsai and Coyle 1995). In schizophrenia, reduced NAA in PFC has been shown to predict abnormalities in dopamine

metabolism (Bertolino et al. 2000a) and in PFC cortex activation (Bertolino et al. 2000b; Callicott et al. 2000b). We have used this information as an additional criterion to validate the connection between abnormal functional-imaging findings and underlying pathology, assuming that pathology-specific findings should correlate with NAA measures. For example, we found evidence for reduced efficiency (increased activation) in the PFC and other regions within the WM network (e.g., parietal cortex, hippocampus, and anterior cingulate cortex) when comparing schizophrenic patients to healthy comparison subjects (Callicott et al. 2000b). However, only reduced efficiency of the PFC was predicted by NAA measures from that region.

Fletcher et al. (1998) were the first to use a dynamic approach in a study of word recall in schizophrenic patients. Using ^{15}O-H$_2$O blood-flow PET imaging, they found that as word list length increased control subjects increased PFC activation. While patients initially increased PFC activation within a range of performance similar to that of control subjects, PFC blood flow fell at longer list lengths, where patient performance was impaired. These data suggest that control subjects and schizophrenic patients operate on similar activation curves, except that the patient curve declines prior to that of control subjects. We chose the N-back WM task because of its simplicity and ease of conversion to a parametric task (Callicott et al. 2000b). Subjects are asked to recall stimuli seen N previously, with N (and thus WM difficulty) increasing linearly. We chose a group of higher-functioning schizophrenic subjects who were able to maintain reasonable (though impaired) WM performance and sought to map their PFC response at mild and moderate WM impairment. Previously we had found reduced PFC function in the setting of severe WM impairment (Callicott et al. 1998b). We hypothesized that an abnormal physiological response should be present at every level of WM difficulty at which patients showed a behavioral deficit. Also, we predicted that disease-dependent functional findings should be related to in vivo neuronal integrity (NAA measures). We found that patients performed reasonably well at one back and two back (i.e., ~86% correct at 1B and ~80% correct at 2B). Using statistical parametric mapping (SPM96), we looked for regions in which the transition from no back (identifying the stimulus currently seen) to one back and then to two back differed between groups.

Surprisingly, we found evidence for an exaggerated PFC fMRI response in spite of impaired performance. We interpreted this exaggerated response as fundamentally inefficient: patients used greater PFC resources to achieve lesser WM output. Only dorsal PFC NAA measures were correlated with the fMRI response, and this in a negative fashion: reduced NAA (greater neuronal pathology) predicted greater exaggerated PFC fMRI response. Finally, we found a fundamental distinction in the relationship between performance and the PFC fMRI response for control subjects versus patients. In these control subjects, as in a prior sample (Callicott et al. 1999), better performance was associated with greater PFC activation. In patients, however, *worse* performance was associated with greater PFC activation, with poor performers (with lower PFC NAA) exhibiting the greatest loss in PFC efficiency. The major drawback to this study was the fact that we did not cover a large enough portion of the load-response curve; thus we did not find portions of the curve over which patients and control subjects performed and activated similarly, nor a portion over which patients performed poorly and activated less. Nonetheless, we have demonstrated the feasibility of a dynamic design and the utility of concomitant ^{1}H-MRSI measures to assess abnormal findings. Clearly, patients' increased PFC activation at diminished performance levels similar to those attained by control subjects at higher N back—levels where control subjects *decrease* PFC activation—establishes the existence of separate curves for patients and control subjects. Armed with enough points to establish true curves, one could address on an individual and group basis the question of whether interventions such as medication fundamentally improve or worsen cognitive function. With only one point on the curve, functional imaging differences may represent movement up and down the same performance activation curve (an effect unlikely to represent fundamental change in underlying physiology) or may represent fundamental deviation due to a static or ongoing pathophysiological state (see Figure 1–1).

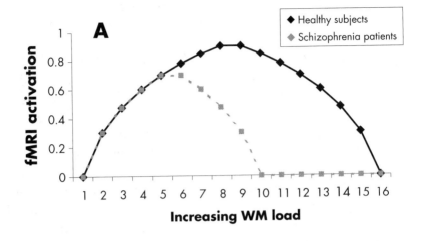

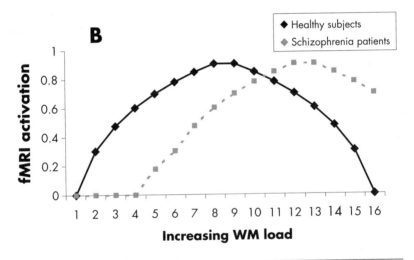

Figure 1–1. Hypothetical working memory (WM) activation curves. **A.** On this hypothesis, both groups operate on a similarly shaped physiological response curve. However, patients show reduced capacity and their activation curve falls at lower WM load. Depending upon which portion of the curve is mapped, patients may show activation equal to that of control subjects or less (i.e., hypofrontality). **B.** In contrast, patients operate on fundamentally distinct physiological WM activation curve. Depending upon the portion of the curve examined, patients may have equal activation, reduced activation (e.g., hypofrontality), or increased activation (e.g., hyperfrontality). Apparently contradictory results could be obtained if the physiological response were not examined over a wide range of WM loads.

Magnetic Resonance and Genetic Susceptibility

We have reviewed the use of dynamic functional brain mapping as an adjunct to clinical management and assessment. For reasons already discussed, fMRI is not likely to produce diagnostic information in the near future. However, functional brain imaging will identify individuals in whom neurophysiological response to cognitive stress deviates significantly from normal. The identification of these outliers, while not diagnostic, offers an alternative classification system that may prove a valuable tool in the identification of genetic susceptibility to mental illness (intermediate or endophenotypic). Schizophrenia and other major mental disorders clearly have a heritable component but like adult-onset diabetes and hypertension do not appear to be the result of one gene. Rather they are products of multiple genes interacting with environmental stressors to produce manifest illness (Kidd 1997; O'Rourke et al. 1982; Risch and Merikangas 1996). In contradistinction to Mendelian disorders such as Huntington's disease, each of several genes may contribute only a small amount of variance to the overall susceptibility to mental illness and may interact in a complex fashion (epistasis). This is illustrated by our COMT finding in which the COMT genotype is clearly associated with schizophrenia but may introduce only 5% of the variance in the prefrontal function (M.F. Egan et al., unpublished observations, 2000).

The difficulty of identifying these multiple genes is further complicated by the imprecision of clinical phenotypes used to identify affected individuals, as typified by DSM-IV criteria (American Psychiatric Association 1994; Crowe 1993). However, the identification of fundamental characteristics strongly associated with schizophrenia in some susceptible families is a useful alternative classification system for linkage or association studies. Correctly ascertained, functional imaging abnormalities in schizophrenic patients and their relatives may be particularly useful, since they presumably lie closer to gene function than clinical diagnoses that may reflect the interaction of several pathological processes (Cannon et al. 1994). In other complex disorders, the endophenotype approach has been used with success. Using subclinical electroencephalogram (EEG) abnormalities as the endophenotype, Greenberg et al. (1988) were able to find linkage on chromosome 6 to juvenile myoclonic epilepsy. In schizophrenia, more traditional intermediate phenotypes include eye-tracking dysfunction (Holzman et al. 1984; Siever and Coursey 1985), neuropsychological measures such as WM capacity (Franke et al. 1992; Goldberg et al. 1990), and abnormal auditory P50 evoked potentials (Siegel et al. 1984). This approach has already generated several findings in schizophrenia. Using abnormal P50 inhibition as the intermediate phenotype, Freedman et al. (1997) found linkage in nine multiplex families to a locus on chromosome 15 (15q13–14) near the α 7-nicotinic cholinergic receptor gene. Shihabuddin et al. (1996) linked a marker on chromosome 5 (5p14.1–13.1) to increased ventricular size and frontal-parietal atrophy. Finally, Arolt et al. (1996) found linkage of eye-tracking dysfunction to two regions on the short arm of chromosome 6.

The likelihood that a particular endophenotype is significantly heritable can be estimated using a relative risk statistic (Risch 1990). Relative risk (λ_s) is computed by determining the frequency of the given phenotype in siblings of ill probands as compared to its frequency in the general population. Since siblings share on average 50% of their ill sibling's genes, siblings will be more likely to inherit some of the risk genes (even if they are unaffected by mental illness) than the general public, and having these genes they will be more likely than the general public to express endophenotypes. Relative risk greater than 2 (i.e., twice the expression of a phenotype in siblings as opposed to a control population) is considered the critical threshold.

Using ^{1}H-MRSI, we reported the first functional neuroimaging phenotype shared by schizophrenic patients and their unaffected siblings (Callicott et al. 1998a). In a sample of 47 schizophrenic patients, 60 unaffected siblings, and 66 healthy control subjects, we found that decreased neuronal function in the hippocampal area (reduced NAA measures) was approximately 4–8 times more common among siblings than among control subjects (λ_s = 3.8–8.8). As was done in the studies noted above, we generated a qualitative phenotype (i.e., NAA measure < one standard deviation away from normal) from a quantitative measure (i.e., NAA). When treated as a quantitative measure, NAA measures showed a low predictive value between patients and their siblings (intraclass correlation = 0.12).

While ^{1}H-MRSI is reasonably reliable within individuals over time (Bertolino et al. 1998b), there may still be too much noise in present techniques to produce a reliable quantitative trait that could be used in a quantitative trait locus analysis. In addition, PFC inefficiency during WM also appears to be overrepresented in unaffected siblings of schizophrenic patients (Callicott et al., unpublished observations, 1999). We used echo-planar functional MRI and a parametric N-back WM task to search for abnormal physiological characteristics in unaffected siblings of schizophrenic patients ($n = 25$), and healthy control subjects ($n = 15$). Unaffected siblings and healthy control subjects performed with similar accuracy. However, unaffected siblings were significantly hyperfrontal (similar to their schizophrenic siblings) in spite of working memory accuracy equal to that of control subjects. We replicated this finding using a separate cohort of siblings ($n = 29$) and control subjects ($n = 24$) using a different fMRI design (spiral pulse sequence and periodic design) and a 2-back WM task.

Conclusions

Functional MRI and ^{1}H-MRSI represent significant technical advances for functional neuroimaging. However, the clinical applicability of both methodologies remains to be seen. In particular, fMRI is not more likely than its predecessors to provide pathognomonic findings for diagnostic purposes. Rather, the use of dynamic designs may provide useful functional characterization of putatively affected brain regions in psychiatric illness. As with cardiac stress tests, these fMRI stress tests may be most useful at providing quantifiable measures of function that may be used to guide treatment and assist prognostication. ^{1}H-MRSI is particularly valuable in that it provides the only in vivo measure of neuronal pathology (or health) via NAA measures. Both fMRI and ^{1}H-MRSI are able to characterize populations on the basis of statistical deviation from normal. This characterization of key cortical functions as neuroimaging endophenotypes may provide a solution to the quandary presented by the genetic complexity of mental illness. The development of fMRI techniques continues at a rapid pace, particularly utilizing the increased power of high-field magnets (e.g., 3 T) and exploring novel applications such as diffusion tensor imaging (Buchsbaum et al. 1998). Based on past experience, however, these developments will be most useful if designed with an eye toward quantification of neuropathology rather than toward novel pathognomonic findings.

References

Abrams R, Taylor MA: Differential EEG patterns in affective disorder and schizophrenia. Arch Gen Psychiatry 36(12):1355–1358, 1979

Akbarian S, Sucher NJ, Bradley D, et al: Selective alterations in gene expression for NMDA receptor subunits in prefrontal cortex of schizophrenics. J Neurosci 16(1):19–30, 1996

American Psychiatric Association: Diagnostic and Statistical Manual of Mental Disorders, 4th Edition. Washington, DC, American Psychiatric Association, 1994

Arnold SE, Gur RE, Shapiro RM, et al: Prospective clinicopathologic studies of schizophrenia: accrual and assessment of patients. Am Psychiatry 152(5):731–737, 1995

Arolt V, Lencer R, Nolte A, et al: Eye tracking dysfunction is a putative phenotypic susceptibility marker of schizophrenia and maps to a locus on chromosome 6p in families with multiple occurrence of the disease. Am J Med Genet 67:564–579, 1996

Benes FM, Davidson B, Bird ED: Quantitative cytoarchitectural studies of the cerebral cortex of schizophrenics. Arch Gen Psychiatry 43:31–35, 1986

Benes FM, McSparren J, Bird ED, et al: Deficits in small interneurons in prefrontal and cingulate cortices of schizophrenic and schizoaffective patients. Arch Gen Psychiatry 48(11):996–1001, 1991

Bertolino A, Nawroz S, Mattay VS, et al: Regionally specific pattern of neurochemical pathology in schizophrenia as assessed by multislice proton magnetic resonance spectroscopic imaging. Am J Psychiatry 153(12):1554–1563, 1996

Bertolino A, Callicott JH, Ellman I, et al: Regionally specific neuronal pathology in untreated patients with schizophrenia: a proton magnetic resonance spectroscopic imaging study. Biol Psychiatry 43(9):641–648, 1998a

Bertolino A, Callicott, JH, Nawroz S, et al: Reproducibility of proton magnetic resonance spectroscopic imaging in patients with schizophrenia. Neuropsychopharmacology 18:1–8, 1998b

Bertolino A, Brier A, Callicott JH, et al: The relationship between dorsolateral prefrontal neuronal N-acetylaspartate and evoked release of striatal dopamine in schizophrenia. Neuropsychopharmacology 22:125–132, 2000a

Bertolino A, Esposito G, Callicott JH, et al: Specific relationship between prefrontal neuronal N-acetylaspartate and activation of the working memory cortical network in schizophrenia. Am J Psychiatry 157(1): 26–33, 2000b

Bogerts B, Falkai P, Greve B, et al: The neuropathology of schizophrenia: past and present. J Hirnforsch 34(2):193–205, 1993

Braus DF, Ende G, Weber-Fahr W, et al: Antipsychotic drug effects on motor activation measured by functional magnetic resonance imaging in schizophrenic patients. Schizophr Res 39(1):19–29, 1999

Braus DF, Ende G, Hubrich-Ungureanu P, et al: Cortical response to motor stimulation in neuroleptic-naive first episode schizophrenics. Psychiatry Res 98(3):145–54, 2000

Breiter HC, Rauch SL, Kwong KK, et al: Functional magnetic resonance imaging of symptom provocation in obsessive-compulsive disorder. Arch Gen Psychiatry 53:595–606, 1996

Breiter HC, Gollub RL, Weisskoff RM, et al: Acute effects of cocaine on human brain activity and emotion. Neuron 19:591–611, 1997

Buchsbaum MS, Tang CY, Peled S, et al: MRI white matter diffusion anisotropy and PET metabolic rate in schizophrenia. Neuroreport 9(3):425–30, 1998

Buckley PF, Friedman L, Wu D, et al: Functional magnetic resonance imaging in schizophrenia: initial methodology and evaluation of the motor cortex. Psychiatry Research: Neuroimaging 74:13–23, 1997

Bullmore E, Brammer M, Williams SC, et al: Functional MR imaging of confounded hypofrontality. Hum Brain Mapp 8(2–3):86–91, 1999

Callicott JH, Egan MF, Bertolino A, et al: Hippocampal N-acetylaspartate in unaffected siblings of patients with schizophrenia: a possible intermediate neurobiological phenotype [published erratum appears in Biol Psychiatry 1999 Jan 15;45(2):following 244]. Biol Psychiatry 44(10):941–50, 1998a

Callicott JH, Ramsey NF, Tallent K, et al: Functional magnetic resonance imaging brain mapping in psychiatry: methodological issues illustrated in a study of working memory in schizophrenia. Neuropsychopharmacology 18:186–196, 1998b

Callicott JH, Mattay VS, Bertolino A, et al: Physiological characteristics of capacity constraints in working memory as revealed by functional MRI. Cerebral Cortex 9(1): 20–26, 1999

Callicott JH, Bertolino A, Egan MF, et al: A selective relationship between prefrontal N-acetylaspartate measures and negative symptoms in schizophrenia. Am J Psychiatry 157(10):1646–1651, 2000a

Callicott JH, Bertolino A, Mattay VS, et al: Physiological dysfunction of the dorsolateral prefrontal cortex in schizophrenia revisited. Cereb Cortex 10:1078–1092, 2000b

Cannon MD, Zorrilla LE, Shtasel D, et al: Neuropsychological functioning in siblings discordant for schizophrenia and healthy volunteers. Arch Gen Psychiatry 51:651–661, 1994

Carter CS, Perlstein W, Ganguli R, et al: Functional hypofrontality and working memory dysfunction in schizophrenia. Am J Psychiatry 155(9):1285–1287, 1998

Cecil KM, Lenkinski RE, Gur RE, et al: Proton magnetic resonance spectroscopy in the frontal and temporal lobes of neuroleptic naive patients with schizophrenia. Neuropsychopharmacology 20(2):131–140, 1999

Cohen BM, Yurgelun-Todd D, English CD, et al: Abnormalities of regional distribution of cerebral vasculature in schizophrenia detected by dynamic susceptibility contrast MRI. Am J Psychiatry 152(12): 1801–1803, 1995

Crowe RR: Candidate genes in psychiatry: an epidemiological perspective. Am J Med Genet 48:74–77, 1993

Curtis VA, Bullmore ET, Brammer MJ, et al: Attenuated frontal activation during a verbal fluency task in patients with schizophrenia. Am J Psychiatry 155(8):1056–1063, 1998

Curtis VA, Bullmore ET, Morris RG, et al: Attenuated frontal activation in schizophrenia may be task dependent. Schizophr Res 37(1):35–44, 1999

David AS, Woodruff PW, Howard R, et al: Auditory hallucinations inhibit exogenous activation of auditory association cortex. Neuroreport 7(4):932–936, 1996

Dierks T, Linden DE, Jandl M, et al: Activation of Heschl's gyrus during auditory hallucinations. Neuron 22(3):615–621, 1999

Fletcher PC, McKenna PJ, Frith CD, et al: Brain activations in schizophrenia during a graded memory task studied with functional neuroimaging. Arch Gen Psychiatry 55(11):1001–1008, 1998

Franke P, Maier W, Hain C, et al: Wisconsin card sorting test: an indicator of vulnerability to schizophrenia? Schizophr Res 6(3):243–249, 1992

Franzen G, Ingvar DH: Abnormal distribution of cerebral activity in chronic schizophrenia. J Psychiatr Res 12(3):199–214, 1975

Freedman R, Coon H, Myles-Worsley M, et al: Linkage of a neurophysiological deficit in schizophrenia to a chromosome 15 locus. Proc Natl Acad Sci U S A 94(2):587–592, 1997

Frith CD, Friston KJ, Herold S, et al: Regional brain activity in chronic schizophrenic patients during the performance of a verbal fluency task. Br J Psychiatry 167(3):343–349, 1995

Funahashi S, Bruce CJ, Goldman-Rakic PS et al: Mnemonic coding of visual space in the monkey's dorsolateral prefrontal cortex. J Neurophysiol 61(2):331–349, 1989

Funahashi S, Bruce CJ, Goldman-Rakic PS: Neuronal activity related to saccadic eye movements in the monkey's dorsolateral prefrontal cortex. J Neurophysiol 65(6):1464–1483, 1991

Gevins AS, Morgan NH, Bressler SL, et al: Human neuroleptic patterns predict performance accuracy. Science 235(4788):580–585, 1987

Goldberg TE, Ragland JD, Torrey EF, et al: Neuropsychological assessment of monozygotic twins discordant for schizophrenia. Arch Gen Psychiatry 47:1066–1072, 1990

Goldberg TE, Berman KF, Fleming K, et al: Uncoupling cognitive workload and prefrontal cortical physiology: a PET rCBF study. Neuroimage 7(4 Pt 1):296–303, 1998

Greenberg DA, Delgado-Escueta AV, Widelitz H, et al: Juvenile myoclonic epilepsy (JME) may be linked to the BF and HLA loci on human chromosome 6. Am J Med Genet 31(1):185–192, 1988

Holzman PS, Proctor LR, Hughes DW: Eye-tracking patterns in schizophrenia. Science 181(95):179–181, 1973

Holzman PS, Solomon CM, Levin S, et al: Pursuit eye movement dysfunction in schizophrenia: family evidence for specificity. Arch Gen Psychiatry 41:136–139, 1984

Ingvar D, Franzen, G: Distribution of cerebral activity in chronic schizophrenia. Lancet 2:1484–1486, 1974

Jenkins BG, Klivenyi P, Kustermann E, et al: Nonlinear decrease over time in N-acetylaspartate levels in the absence of neuronal loss and increases in glutamine and glucose in transgenic Huntington's disease mice. J Neurochem 74(5):2108–2119, 2000

Kidd KK: Can we find genes for schizophrenia? Am J Med Genet 74: 104–111, 1997

Kraepelin E: Dementia Praecox and Paraphrenia (1912). Translated by Barclay RM. Edinburgh, E. & S. Livingstone, 1971

Levin JM, Ross MH, Renshaw PF: Clinical applications of functional MRI in neuropsychiatry. J Neuropsychiatry Clin Neurosci 7(4):511–522, 1995

Maas LC, Lukas SE, Kaufman MJ, et al: Functional magnetic resonance imaging of human brain activation during cue-induced cocaine craving. Am J Psychiatry 155:124–126, 1998

Mannisto PT, Kaakkola S: Catechol O-methyltransferase (COMT): biochemistry, molecular biology, pharmacology, and clinical efficacy of the new selective COMT inhibitors. Pharmacol Rev 51(4):593–628, 1999

Manoach DS, Press DZ, Thangaraj V, et al: Schizophrenic subjects activate dorsolateral prefrontal cortex during a working memory task, as measured by fMRI. Biol Psychiatry 45(9):1128–1137, 1999

Manoach DS, Gollub RL, Benson ES, et al: Schizophrenic subjects show aberrant fMRI activation of dorsolateral prefrontal cortex and basal ganglia during working memory performance [In Process Citation]. Biol Psychiatry 48(2):99–109, 2000

Mattay VS, Callicott JH, Bertolino A, et al: Abnormal functional lateralization of the sensorimotor cortex in patients with schizophrenia. Neuroreport 8(13):2977–2984, 1997

Mellers JD, Adachi N, Takei N, et al: SPET study of verbal fluency in schizophrenia and epilepsy. Br J Psychiatry 173:69–74, 1998

Northoff G, Braus DF, Sartorius A, et al: Reduced activation and altered laterality in two neuroleptic-naive catatonic patients during a motor task in functional MRI. Psychol Med 29:997–1002, 1999

O'Rourke DH, Gottesman II, Suarez BK, et al: Refutation of the general single-locus model for the etiology of schizophrenia. Am J Hum Genet 34(4):630–649, 1982

Phillips ML, Williams L, Senior C, et al: A differential neural response to threatening and non-threatening negative facial expressions in paranoid and non-paranoid schizophrenics. Psychiatric Research: Neuroimaging 92(8):11–31, 1999

Piercy M: The effects of cerebral lesions on intellectual function: a review of current research trends. Br J Psychiatry 110:310–352, 1964

Ragland JD, Gur RC, Glahn DC, et al: Frontotemporal cerebral blood flow change during executive and declarative memory tasks in schizophrenia: a positron emission tomography study. Neuropsychology 12(3):399–413, 1998

Rajkowska G, Selemon LD, Goldman-Rakic PS, et al: Neuronal and glial somal size in the prefrontal cortex: a postmortem morphometric study of schizophrenia and Huntington disease. Arch Gen Psychiatry 55(3):215–224, 1998

Renshaw PF, Yurgelun-Todd DA, Cohen BM, et al: Greater hemodynamic response to photic stimulation in schizophrenic patients: an echo planar MRI study. Am J Psychiatry 151(10):1493–1495, 1994

Risch N: Linkage strategies for genetically complex traits, II: the power of affected relative pairs. Am J Hum Genet 46(2):229–241, 1990

Risch N, Merikangas K, et al: The future of genetic studies of complex human diseases. Science 273:1516–1517, 1996

Schneider F, Weiss U, Kessler C, et al: Differential amygdala activation in schizophrenia during sadness. Schizophr Res 34(3):133–142, 1998

Schroder J, Wenz F, Schad LR, et al: Sensorimotor cortex and supplementary motor area changes in schizophrenia: a study with functional magnetic resonance imaging. Br J Psychiatry 167(2):197–201, 1995

Schroder J, Essig M, Baudendistel K, et al: Motor dysfunction and sensorimotor cortex activation changes in schizophrenia: a study with functional magnetic resonance imaging. Neuroimage 9(1):81–87, 1999

Selemon LD, Rajkowska G, Goldman-Rakic PS: Abnormally high neuronal density in the schizophrenic cortex: a morphometric analysis of prefrontal area 9 and occipital area 17. Arch Gen Psychiatry 52:805–818, 1995

Selemon LD, Rajkowska G, Goldman-Rakic PS: Elevated neuronal density in prefrontal area 46 in brains from schizophrenic patients: application of a three-dimensional, stereologic counting method. J Comp Neurol 392(3):402–412, 1998

Shihabuddin L, Silverman JM, Buchsbaum MS, et al: Ventricular enlargement associated with linkage marker for schizophrenia-related disorders in one pedigree. Molecular Psychiatry 1:215–222, 1996

Siegel C, Waldo M, Mizner G, et al: Deficits in sensory gating in schizophrenic patients and their relatives. Arch Gen Psychiatry 41:607–612, 1984

Siever LJ, Coursey RD: Biological markers for schizophrenia and the biological high-risk approach. J Nerv Ment Dis 173(1):4–16, 1985

Stevens AA, Goldman-Rakic PS, Gore JC, et al: Cortical dysfunction in schizophrenia during auditory word and tone working memory demonstrated by functional magnetic resonance imaging. Arch Gen Psychiatry 55(12):1097–1103, 1998

Tauscher J, Fischer P, Neumeister A, et al: Low frontal electroencephalographic coherence in neuroleptic-free schizophrenic patients. Biol Psychiatry 44(6):438–447, 1998

Taylor S, Tandon R, Koeppe R: PET study of greater visual activation in schizophrenia. Am J Psychiatry 154:1296–1298, 1997

Thomas MA, Ke Y, Levitt J, et al: Preliminary study of frontal lobe 1H MR spectroscopy in childhood-onset schizophrenia. J Magn Reson Imaging 8(4):841–846, 1998

Tsai G, Coyle JT: N-acetylaspartate in neuropsychiatric disorders. Prog Neurobiol 46(5):531–540, 1995

Volz H, Gaser C, Hager F, et al: Decreased frontal activation in schizophrenics during stimulation with the Continuous Performance Test: a functional magnetic resonance imaging study. Eur Psychiatry 14(1):17–24, 1999

Weinberger DR, Berman KF: Prefrontal function in schizophrenia: confounds and controversies. Phil Trans Royal Soc Med 351:1495–1503, 1996

Weinberger DR, Berman KF, Illowsky BP: Physiological dysfunction of dorsolateral prefrontal cortex in schizophrenia, III: a new cohort and evidence for a monoaminergic mechanism. Arch Gen Psychiatry 45(7):609–615, 1988

Weinberger DR, Berman KF, Suddath R, et al: Evidence for dysfunction of a prefrontal-limbic network in schizophrenia: an MRI and rCBF study of discordant monozygotic twins. Am J Psychiatry 149:890–897, 1992

Weinberger DR, Mattay V, Callicott JH, et al: fMRI applications in schizophrenia research. Neuroimage 4(3 Pt 3):S118–S126, 1996

Wenz F, Schad LR, Knopp MV, et al: Functional magnetic resonance imaging at 1.5 T: activation pattern in schizophrenic patients receiving neuroleptic medication. Magn Reson Med 12:975–982, 1994

Woo TU, Whitehead RE, Melchitzky DS, et al: A subclass of prefrontal gamma-aminobutyric acid axon terminals are selectively altered in schizophrenia. Proc Natl Acad Sci U S A 95(9):5341–5346, 1998

Woodruff PWR, Wright IC, Bullmore ET, et al: Auditory hallucinations and the temporal cortical response to speech in schizophrenia: a functional magnetic resonance imaging study. Am J Psychiatry 154:1676–1682, 1997

Yurgelun-Todd DA, Waternaux CM, Cohen BM, et al: Functional magnetic resonance imaging of schizophrenic patients and comparison subjects during word production. Am J Psychiatry 153(2):200–205, 1996

Chapter 2

Cognitive Neuroscience

The New Neuroscience of the Mind and Its Implications for Psychiatry

Cameron S. Carter, M.D.

Over the past several years there has been a remarkable surge of interest in the role that deficits in cognition might play in the disability associated with common mental disorders. In the study of schizophrenia, for example, it has become increasingly clear that cognitive deficits—in particular disturbances of attention and memory—are the strongest predictor of functional outcome, far more so than positive and negative symptoms (Green 1996).

In parallel with these developments, a whole new field of neuroscience—*cognitive* neuroscience—has emerged, and rapid advances have been made in our understanding of the neural basis of human cognition. This field focuses on how cells and systems in the brain interact to perform specific cognitive functions. Cognitive neuroscience emerged as cognitive psychologists became interested in how cognitive functions such as attention and memory are implemented in the brain (e.g., Gazzaniga et al. 1998; Posner and Petersen 1990) at the same time that physiologists interested in the functional significance of brain activity at the single neuron level began using cognitive psychological methods and theories to advance their research (Fuster 1988; Goldman-Rakic 1991). Just as these two communities began to interact, remarkable advances were made in neurophysiological techniques for measuring brain activity in humans during cognitive task performance. These developments led to the application of positron emission tomography (PET), cortical evoked potentials (ERPs), magnetoencephalography, and, more recently, functional magnetic resonance imaging (fMRI) in studies of the neural basis of cognition in healthy humans. As a result of these studies, remarkable progress has been made understanding the circuitry, patterns of neuronal firing, and computational properties of neural systems underlying normal perception, attention, memory, and language-related functions.

The goal of cognitive neuroscience is to build an understanding of brain–behavior relationships based upon converging data across multiple levels of analysis. Hence our interpretation of functional neuroimaging data is constrained by our understanding (from cognitive psychology) of the cognitive processes being examined, by data from studies of human subjects with known lesions in the brain, and by data from animal research. The latter studies typically use single or population neuron recording, focal lesions, or pharmacological manipulations in nonhuman primates or other species performing cognitive tasks. This integration of data from multiple sources has rapidly expanded our understanding of the neural basis of cognition. The unprecedented opportunity for clinical neuroscience is to take this body of knowledge and build upon it, using methodologies such as functional neuroimaging, to develop an understanding of the neural basis of cognitive impairments in mental disorders. Since these cognitive impairments are typically not only disabling but also treatment-refractory, the insights obtained by this approach promise to facilitate the development of more effective therapies, which may reduce the burden of disability for our patients.

Cognitive neuroscience–based imaging approaches may also permit the development of clinical brain-imaging tools to facilitate the diagnostic process early in the course of psychiatric disorders, when ascertainment may currently be impossible, as during the prodromal phase of schizophrenia or early in the course of dementia. Such clinical imaging tools may also one day provide a means to predict and track the effects of specific treatments for impaired cognition in psychiatric disorders.

In this chapter I will discuss the cognitive neuroscience's far-reaching implications for research into the pathophysiology of mental disorders. In particular, I will describe how new, cognitive neuroscience–based functional imaging studies may help to clarify some ambiguities arising out of the initial wave of functional imaging studies of mental disorders. I will begin with a neural-systems model of executive functions developed in our laboratory. The term *executive functions* refers to the set of cognitive operations required to maintain organized information and coordinated actions in the brain. The neural systems supporting executive control appear to be uniquely sensitive to the effects of psychiatric disease. A detailed account of the contributions of subregions of the frontal cortex to executive functions, based on recent event-related fMRI studies performed in our laboratory, will be described, together with a discussion of how abnormal physiology in these regions is likely to be associated with two common serious mental disorders, schizophrenia—a disorder of *under*control—and obsessive-compulsive disorder (OCD)—a disorder of *over*control.

Executive Functions and the Brain

Imagine that you are driving your car home from work. You come to an intersection and the light is red. Just as you begin to slow down, you notice that a policeman is in the center of the intersection waving traffic ahead vigorously. You realize that you have no recollection of driving through several heavily trafficked intersections, having been lost in thought about the day's events. Despite the life-threatening dangers of being at the wheel of a car, your actions under these circumstances have been quite routine, requiring little or no attention. Your initial response to the red light is to stop, but after slowing momentarily you quickly accelerate through the intersection as directed by the officer. How were you able to flexibly adjust your attention to emerge from your reverie and respond so seamlessly to such an ambiguous set of environmental demands? The domain of human cognition associated with these amazingly fluid adjustments of attention is referred to as *executive functions*.

Cognitive models of executive functions (e.g., Carter et al. 1999) generally distinguish between *strategic* functions—those involved in top-down control, representing goals and allocating attention in a task-appropriate manner (ignore the traffic light and pay attention to the policeman!)—and *evaluative* or performance-monitoring functions, which indicate the degree to which controlled processing must be engaged (stop daydreaming and pay attention to driving!). A schematic model of executive functions, illustrating the interactive nature of top-down control and performance monitoring, is shown in Figure 2–1.

A large, convergent set of data from cognitive neuroscience implicates the frontal lobes in playing a central role in executive functions. Two frontal regions in particular have been emphasized: 1) the anterior cingulate cortex (ACC), on the medial surface of the brain (astride the corpus callosum), and 2) the dorsolateral prefrontal cortex (DLPFC), on the lateral convexity. Previous human functional-imaging studies have shown that when executive control is engaged both regions become more active (D'Esposito et al. 1995; Posner and Petersen 1990; Smith and Jonides 1999). However, recent studies by our group and others suggest that, while both regions are active under conditions that require high levels of control, they contribute unique, complementary functions.

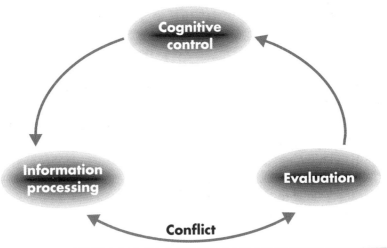

Figure 2–1. A schematic model of executive functions as a set of dynamic processes. Cognitive control mechanisms, such as attentional set, bias information processing in a task-appropriate manner. Evaluative processes monitor for evidence of poor performance, such as response conflict, and signal when control needs to be more strongly engaged.

ACC and Performance Monitoring

The ACC is composed of a gyral fold and associated sulcus located on the medial surface of the frontal lobe, adjacent to the corpus callosum. This region has rich, bidirectional connections with the association cortex of the DLPFC and parietal, temporal, and entorhinal cortices. It also receives rich projections from the amygdala. The ACC, in particular the cortex in the cingulate sulcus, also has rich efferent connections to multiple levels of the motor system, including the supplementary motor area, premotor and motor cortex, and anterior horn cells of the spinal cord (Dum and Strick 1993; Morecraft et al. 1997). The unique connectivity of this region, along with observations of brain-injured subjects and functional neuroimaging studies, has frequently led to the claim that the ACC is a critical element in the neural system associated with executive processes and behavioral regulation (D'Esposito et al. 1995; Mesulam 1990; Posner and Petersen 1990). However, the precise contribution of this region to this broad class of processes has not been well understood.

Two broad theories of ACC function during executive control have been proposed. The first, based upon the results of functional neuroimaging studies, is that the ACC serves a *strategic* function related to the top-down control of attention. This highly influential theory has been invoked to account for the ACC activity observed in functional brain imaging studies during a wide range of demanding cognitive tasks. One task reliably associated with ACC activation is the Stroop task, in which subjects are required to name the color of a word that is itself the name of a color. This task places particularly high demands on selective attention if the color and the word are different (e.g., if the word RED is printed in blue, referred to as an *incongruent trial*); this is because reading a word is quite automatic, and it is difficult to overcome the tendency to read the word as such rather than to name its physical color. In fact, it appears that both processes are occurring in the brain simultaneously, because subjects are much slower at naming word color in an incongruent trial than when word and color are the same (a *congruent trial*). This longer response time is thought to reflect a process called *response conflict*, the simultaneous activation of incompatible responses. Early interpretations of ACC activation during the Stroop task proposed that it reflects the engagement of top-down control to allocate attention toward the color and away from the word, reducing conflict and enhancing response speed (e.g., Pardo et al. 1991).

The second (perhaps less well-known) theory of ACC function derives from electrophysiological studies of the error-related negativity (ERN; see Figure 2–2), a scalp potential recorded during ERP that appears to have its source in the ACC (Dehaene et al. 1994; Falkenstein et al. 1991; Gehring et al. 1993). The ERN is observed concurrent with the execution of an incorrect response on a range of speeded response tasks. ERNs are also observed when subjects make *partial errors*, that is, when subjects begin to make an error but then correct themselves. Several aspects of the ERN, including the observation that the largest ERNs are generated by partial errors and that reaction times on subsequent trials are longer when ERNs are larger, suggest that the ACC is part of a circuit involved in error detection and compensation (Gehring et al. 1993). In other words, this theory proposes that the ACC performs an *evaluative* function in the service of executive control. In an event-related fMRI study (Carter et al. 1998), we showed that when subjects made an error the ACC did show an increase in activity, which is consistent with error-related activity in this region of the brain. However, the same region of the ACC also showed activity during correct trials in which there was response conflict. This suggests that the ACC does not detect errors per se, which would require some rather complicated comparator process by which it somehow has knowledge of what the correct response *should* have been as well the actual, incorrect response being executed. Rather, it simply detects conflict between incompatible response tendencies. On this view, error-related activity would simply reflect conflict between the incorrect response that has just been executed and an ongoing attempt to execute the correct response as subjects continue to attempt to perform as instructed. This has led to an alternative view regarding the evaluative function of the ACC, namely, that this region of the brain detects processing conflicts and thus is part of an error *prevention* network (Carter et al. 1998, 1999). Within this framework, the ACC contributes to executive control by continuously evaluating the level of response conflict in the brain; when it is high, it signals other components of the executive network that attention needs to be more strongly engaged in order to avoid making errors. In terms of our example from everyday life, the ACC would become activated when conflicting stimuli (red light, police officer) suggest conflicting responses (stop, drive on). The ACC would then signal other components of the executive network to pay attention; the executive network would resolve the conflict by retrieving the rule "officer's signal supersedes stop light," ignoring the traffic light, and responding to the officer.

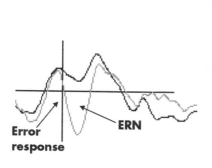 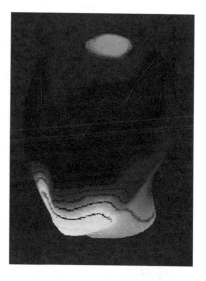

Figure 2–2. The error-related negativity (ERN) is a negative deflection of the surface electroencephalogram (EEG) seen in response-aligned data as subjects make an error. It is maximal at electrodes over medial frontal sites, and dipole modeling suggests that it has its source in the anterior cingulate cortex (ACC). Event-related functional magnetic resonance imaging studies have confirmed that the ACC does show error-related activity but also shows activity during correct trials when there is response conflict.

If the ACC is serving an evaluative performance-monitoring function, detecting response conflicts that indicate the performance is going sour, could it also be involved in strategic processes, adjusting attention in the service of conflict resolution, i.e., better performance? We conducted several experiments in which we manipulated the degree of control and the degree of conflict in an orthogonal manner (Carter et al. 2000). We did this by manipulating subjects' expectancies as well as by examining trial-to-trial adjustments of attention (see also Botvinick et al. 1999; MacDonald et al. 2000). In each case we observed that the ACC was most active when top-down control was weakly engaged, performance poor, and conflict high and least active when attention was strongly engaged, performance good, and conflict low. These data suggest that the ACC is not involved directly in top-down control, but rather serves as a performance monitor, detecting response conflict and signaling other components of the executive network that top-down control needs to be more strongly engaged. If the ACC is not involved in top-down control, however, what regions of the brain—in particular, which regions of the frontal cortex—are?

DLPFC and Top-Down Control

An obvious candidate for top-down control contributor is the DLPFC, on the lateral frontal convexity. This region of prefrontal cortex has been implicated for decades in the control of attention and in working memory (the form of short-term memory that allows us to maintain and manipulate a few items of information without committing them to long-term memory). However, the precise role of this region has been controversial. Recent studies have suggested that for memory functions, this region is less involved with storage and more involved with operations that ensure that the information remembered was appropriate to the task instructions, a strategic executive function (Smith and Jonides 1999). Data from single-cell recording studies of primates suggest that neurons in this region show a characteristic pattern of sustained firing when information is held in mind (Goldman-Rakic 1987), which in turn suggests that some information is being maintained or stored through this activity.

How can a sustained pattern of neuronal activity suggestive of storage be reconciled with a strategic process related to executive control? One possibility is that what is being maintained is a representation of the correct pattern of attention allocation to perform the task according to the goal, referred to as an *attentional set* or *context representation*. We tested this hypothesis using event-related fMRI and a modified version of the Stroop task (MacDonald et al. 2000). On each trial, subjects were cued as to whether they would perform the attention-demanding form of the task (color naming) or simply read the word. We scanned these subjects during a preparatory interval between getting their task cue and being presented with the colored word stimulus, and then again as they responded to the colored word (see Figure 2–3). Areas involved in the representation and maintenance of an attentional set should be active during the period when subjects prepare for the stimulus to appear and relatively more active when they prepare to color-name than to word-read, as the attentional demands are much higher for color naming. The DLPFC was the only region in the brain that showed this pattern of activity, and the more this region was activated by subjects when they prepared to color-name, the better they performed. This result provides strong evidence for a specific executive function for the DLPFC, which is also consistent with the observation that this region shows sustained cellular activity during working-memory tasks in monkeys (Goldman-Rakic 1987). Interestingly, in this study the ACC did not show preparatory activity but again showed conflict-related activity that correlated with poor performance, consistent with a performance-monitoring function.

This work suggests that unique, complementary functions are implemented in lateral and medial frontal cortex. A specific mapping between the conceptual model shown in Figure 2–1 and these regions is also suggested. The DLPFC shows increased activity associated with increased top-down control via the representation and maintenance of an attentional set, while the ACC evaluates the level of response conflict and signals when control needs to be more strongly engaged. These functions have also been implemented quite successfully in computational models

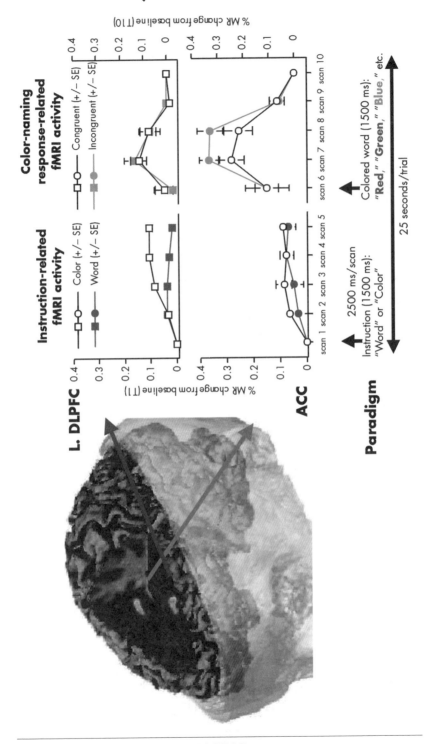

Figure 2–5. Dissociation of strategic from evaluative processes in the frontal cortex. In this experiment subjects performed the Stroop task: that is, were cued to either read or name the color of a colored word that was also the name of a color (e.g., the word RED printed in green ink). The dorsolateral prefrontal cortex (DLPFC) became active after the cue, that is, as subjects prepared to perform the task, and was most active when subjects prepared to perform the difficult (color-naming) version of the task. The anterior cingulate cortex (ACC) showed conflict-related activity during color-naming trials. The DLPFC activation correlated with good task performance, ACC activity correlated with poor performance.

Source. Reprinted with permission from MacDonald AW, Cohen JD, Stenger VA, et al.: "Dissociating the Role of Dorsolateral Prefrontal and Anterior Cingulate Cortex in Cognitive Control." *Science* 288:1835–1838, 2000. Copyright 2000, American Association for the Advancement of Science.

within the parallel distributed processing framework (McClelland and Rumelhart 1986) of executive functions during a range of cognitive tasks (Botvinick et al. 1999); however, a description of this modeling work is beyond the scope of this chapter. We will now extend this framework into clinical neuroscience in an effort to shed light on the pathophysiology of disturbed executive functions in schizophrenia and OCD.

Impaired Executive Functions in Schizophrenia: Role of DLPFC and ACC

Since the earliest descriptions of schizophrenia, cognitive dysfunction has been noted as a prominent aspect of the illness (Bleuler 1911/1950; Kraepelin 1912/1971). For example, Bleuler argued strongly that deficits in the ability to control attention were the underlying basis for the associational disturbances that distinguished schizophrenia from the other psychoses. However, the clinical significance of cognitive deficits in schizophrenia has only recently been systematically examined. In a number of studies, cognitive dysfunction in schizophrenia has been shown to be related to behavioral disorganization (Barch and Carter 1998; Cohen et al. 1999; Green 1998; Liddle and Morris 1991), providing some support for the Bleulerian view. Most importantly, cognitive dysfunction is a strong predictor of poor outcome (Green 1996, 1998; Weinberger and Gallhofer 1997), more robustly so than hallucinations and delusions. Yet cognitive dysfunction shows only modest, if any, improvement with currently available therapies for schizophrenia (Goldberg et al. 1993; Green 1998).

A wide range of cognitive abnormalities have been reported in schizophrenia. In the domain of higher cognitive functions, disturbances have been described in selective attention (Barch et al. 1999; Carter et al. 1992; Cornblatt et al. 1989; Mirsky 1969; Nuechterlein and Dawson 1984), working memory (Carter et al. 1996; Gold et al. 1997; Keefe et al. 1995; Park and Holtzman 1992), episodic memory (Clare et al. 1993; Saykin et al. 1991; Schwartz et al. 1992; Tamlyn et al. 1992), language production (Barch and Berenbaum 1996; Docherty et al. 1988, 1996; Harvey 1983), and comprehension (Condray et al. 1995; Morice and McNichol 1985).

Since executive processes are engaged across the range of higher cognitive functions that are impaired in schizophrenia, a deficit in executive function has served as the basis of the majority of general theories of cognitive dysfunction in schizophrenia (Braff 1993; Carter and Barch 1998; Cohen and Servan-Schreiber 1993; Liddle 1993; Posner and Abdullaev 1996). However, the *specific* abnormality or abnormalities within the executive system in schizophrenia have yet to be defined. Well-articulated theories have emphasized both disturbances in strategic processes (Braff 1993; Calloway and Naghdi 1982; Cohen and Servan-Schreiber 1993; Shakow 1962) and impaired performance monitoring (Feinberg 1978; Frith and Done 1989; Gray et al. 1990; Malenka et al. 1982).

To understand the pathophysiology of schizophrenia and to eventually develop specific treatments for cognitive remediation and disability reduction in schizophrenia, we need to understand the functional brain circuitry associated with impaired cognition. A century before the functional imaging revolution, it was speculated that impaired cognition in schizophrenia might reflect frontal lobe dysfunction. Early reports using PET and other radionuclide-based functional brain imaging methods tended to support this view (Ingvar and Franzen 1974). Over the subsequent decades, many reports and reviews in the literature have shown that hypofrontality is a frequent finding in both medicated and unmedicated schizophrenic patients (e.g., Andreasen et al. 1992; Buchsbaum 1990; Taylor 1996). Hypofrontality is not, however, an invariant feature of schizophrenia (Gur and Gur 1995) and is much more commonly observed when patients are engaged in a cognitive task that activates the frontal lobes in normal subjects (Carter et al. 1998). Both medial and lateral hypofrontality have been reported in schizophrenia in both resting and activation studies, with most findings localizing to the DLPFC and the ACC. Since the vast majority of these studies were conducted at rest or predated the introduction of cognitive neuroscience methodology into psychiatric research, the relationship of altered DLPFC and ACC function to cognitive disability in schizophrenia has been unclear. For example, many previous activation studies used complex tasks that could not isolate the neural correlates of specific cognitive mechanisms. Hence, even though there have now been over 20 years of functional imaging research, and though the data point to alterations in the function of lateral and medial frontal areas associated with executive functions, critical questions remain as to the functional significance of these findings. Is there a selective impairment of DLPFC-related top-down control in schizophrenia, or is the problem an impaired modulation of the DLPFC by the conflict monitoring of the ACC? At present, the data related to this question are unclear, and this is a focus of intense research in our laboratory and others. However, we believe that recent data point to disturbances in both components of the frontal executive network. These findings, and their implications for understanding the pathophysiology of cognitive impairment in schizophrenia, are discussed below.

DLPFC and Impaired Executive Functions in Schizophrenia

Decreased activity in the DLPFC associated with impaired performance of tasks engaging executive functions have been reported for over two decades. Seminal work using the xenon inhalation method by Weinberger and Berman (Weinberger et al. 1986) established during the 1980s that the DLPFC was relatively less active during the Wisconsin Card Sorting Task in schizophrenic patients compared with psychiatrically healthy control subjects. Despite the technical limitations of these studies by contemporary standards, this work was groundbreaking and has served as a benchmark for our ongoing efforts to isolate the neural basis of impaired cognition in schizophrenia. Goldman-Rakic (1987) hypothesized, based on her single-cell recording studies showing that sustained activity in DLPFC correlated with working memory performance in nonhuman primates, that impaired DLPFC activity in schizophrenia was associated with impaired working memory. Working-memory impairment in schizophrenia was subsequently confirmed by a number of investigators using measures of both spatial and verbal working memory (Barch and Carter, 1999; Carter et al. 1996; Cohen and Servan-Schreiber 1993; Keefe 1995; Park and Holzman 1992). Cognitive neuroscientists have increasingly argued that the DLPFC is involved in executive processes governing working memory (Smith and Jonides 1999), and in the event-related fMRI studies described above we have shown that activity in these regions is associated with a specific set of processes related to executive control of working memory and attention, namely, the representation and maintenance of an attentional set. It is within this framework that we now approach the question of the role of the DLPFC in cognitive disability in schizophrenia.

Over the past several years we have investigated the integrity of the DLPFC during working-memory performance in a number of schizophrenic patients at various stages of their illness. In two early studies using ^{15}O-H$_2$O PET, we showed that during a supraspan verbal memory task (Carter et al. 1998; Ganguli et al. 1997) and the N-back working memory task, chronically ill, stable, medicated schizophrenic patients showed significant reductions in DLPFC activation associated with working-memory deficits. More recently, we used fMRI and a parametric version of the N-back task to study a large group of chronic, stable patients treated with a homogeneous regimen of typical neuroleptics. In the N-back tasks, subjects monitor a series of stimuli (in this case letters) and decide whether each word is a repeat of the one presented N previously; for example, for a 2-back task, the target would be A B **A**). In this study, in which we presented multiple levels of N and contrasted the regions that increased as load (N) increased across groups, we confirmed the finding of reduced DLPFC activation and showed that this result was specific to DLPFC; that is, activations in Broca's area and in parietal, motor, and visual areas were normal in patients (see Figure 2–4). Decreased DLPFC activation correlated with both impaired working memory performance and ratings of behavioral disorganization in the patient group.

In a recent study of never-medicated, first-episode schizophrenia (Barch et al., in press) we confirmed that, even at the onset of illness, schizophrenic patients show impaired working-memory–related function in the DLPFC. We used a different task, the AX continuous performance task (AX CPT) to more precisely characterize cognitive mechanisms associated with impaired DLPFC

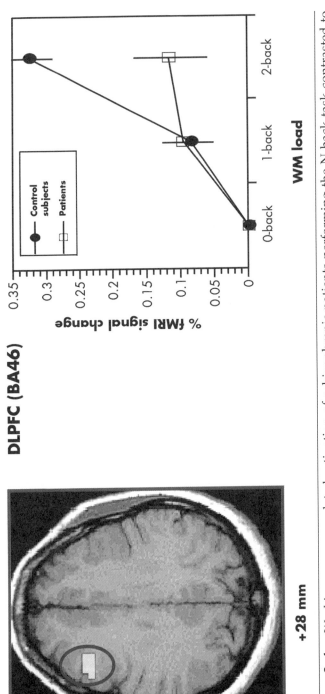

Figure 2–4. Working-memory–related activation of schizophrenic patients performing the N-back task contrasted to that of normal control subjects. While patients and control subjects both showed increased activation in inferior frontal regions with increased working memory demands, schizophrenic patients failed to show this increase in dorsolateral prefrontal cortex (DLPFC). The patients' DLPFC deficit correlated with poor working memory (WM) performance and clinical ratings of behavioral disorganization.

functioning. In this paradigm, subjects must maintain an attentional set across a several-second delay in order to prepare to respond correctly to a probe (the letter X) following a cue (the letter A). We contrasted patients and control subjects on short-delay (0.5 second) and long-delay (9 second) versions of this task and showed that, while both groups activated inferior frontal and parietal regions during the long delay, schizophrenic patients failed to activate the DLPFC. Hence, even during their first episode, prior to treatment schizophrenic patients have an impaired preparatory attentional function of the DLPFC.

ACC and Impaired Performance Monitoring in Schizophrenia

While much of the interest in hypofrontality in schizophrenia has centered on the DLPFC, abnormal ACC activity has also frequently been observed in functional brain imaging studies. Tamminga et al. (1992) reported decreased resting ACC metabolism in a large group of unmedicated schizophrenic patients. Decreased metabolism in the DLPFC and parietal cortex was seen only in the subgroup of patients with the deficit syndrome. Siegel et al. (1993) and Hadnezar et al. (1997) similarly reported extensive cingulate hypometabolism in studies in which subjects performed an auditory CPT (Rosvold et al. 1956) during the uptake phase of the radiotracer. In a study of the relationship between regional brain activity and the symptoms of schizophrenia, resting regional cerebral blood flow in the ACC correlated with patients' levels of disorganization (Liddle et al. 1992). As with the early resting studies suggesting impaired DLPFC function, these resting studies do not speak to the functional significance of impaired ACC activity in schizophrenia.

A number of studies have examined ACC activity in schizophrenia during cognitive activation. During a single positron emission computed tomography (SPECT) study in which unmedicated subjects performed the Tower of London task (a complex planning and problem-solving task), schizophrenic patients showed decreased activity in medial frontal cortex, probably the

ACC (Andreasen et al. 1992). Reduced ACC activation in schizophrenic patients has also been reported during two other tasks involving executive processes, namely, an auditory-verbal supraspan memory task (Ganguli et al. 1997) and paced verbal fluency (Dolan et al. 1995). In each of these studies, the ACC activity seen in control subjects and absent in patients is consistent with an alteration in the evaluative function of this brain region. In a PET blood flow study using the Stroop task for activation, we reported that stable, medicated patients with schizophrenia showed less increase in ACC activity associated with incongruent color-naming trials (Carter et al. 1997).

Further evidence of a disturbance of the performance-monitoring function of the ACC comes from electrophysiological work using the ERN as an index of impaired-performance monitoring in schizophrenia. Kopp and Rist (1999) showed that the ERN was reduced in amplitude in a medicated group of inpatients. This finding has recently been replicated by Ford and colleagues (Mathalon et al. 2000). We have recently used event-related fMRI to investigate error-related activity (indexed by an increase in the fMRI signal during errors) in the ACC and have confirmed that schizophrenic patients show significantly reduced error-related activity in the ACC (Carter et al. 1999).

Could decreased activity in the ACC be secondary to a primary disturbance in the DLPFC in schizophrenia? Since there is rich reciprocal connectivity between the ACC and the DLPFC one could speculate that the ACC is somehow reading out activity arising for the latter region. Recent work from basic cognitive neuroscience suggests that this is unlikely. Patients with focal lesions in the DLPFC have been shown to have an intact ERN (Gehring and Knight 2000). In fact, not only did these frontal-lesioned patients have a normal ERN, but they showed evidence of an ERN-like waveform during correct trials, consistent with the idea that with their impaired attention they will experience more response conflict during task performance. In contrast, when patients with cingulate lesions were studied (Segalowitz et al. 2000), their ERN was absent. Hence, decreased error-related activity in the ACC in schizophrenia appears to reflect a primary disturbance in this region of the brain.

Could the DLPFC activity associated with impaired top-down control be secondary to a primary disturbance in performance monitoring by the ACC? It is possible. Since executive control is a dynamic process and conflict monitoring is likely to be one of the critical mechanisms regulating attention allocation, impaired ACC function would be expected to disrupt the normal modulation of DLPFC activation. However, in studies such as those using fMRI and the N-back and AX CPT tasks described above, where conflict is relatively low, little ACC activation is elicited in control subjects and no significant group differences in this region were observed despite robust decreases in DLPFC activation. Therefore, we believe that it is most likely that the function of both key components of executive control in the frontal cortex is impaired in schizophrenia. This may account for the degree of disorganization present in schizophrenia, which is greater than that seen in patients with focal lesions in either DLPFC or ACC alone. It is also consistent with common abnormalities of markers of local circuit function and disturbed thalamocortical connectivity. In fact, the most robust histopathological finding to date in schizophrenia is a 40% reduction in neurons in the medial dorsal thalamus (Pakkenberg 1990), the source of thalamocortical projections to DLPFC, and this finding has recently been shown to extend to the anterior thalamic nucleus, the primary source of thalamic projections to the ACC (Young et al. 2000). These results suggest a double hit in schizophrenia to the frontal circuitry subserving executive functions.

Overcontrol and Dysfunctional Performance Monitoring in OCD: Role of the ACC

Unlike schizophrenic patients, patients with OCD cannot be characterized as disorganized. In fact, the stereotyped and ritualized behavior of OCD patients can be conceptualized as being *overly* organized. Psychological theories of OCD have drawn upon psychoanalytic theory, learning theory, and recently have also been couched in ethological terms, with obsessional contents and ritualistic behaviors being associated with overactivity in circuitry involving the primitive forebrain (Baxter 1990). In the following paragraphs we will propose a cognitive-neuroscientific hypothesis for certain aspects of OCD symptomatology. Specifically, we will propose that enhanced activity in an ACC-based performance-monitoring function is associated with the doubt, anxiety, and urge to repeat actions that drives compulsive behavior in this illness. This hypothesis is consistent with previous data related to abnormal executive functions in OCD, the results of previous functional imaging studies suggesting hyperactivity in the ACC, the efficacy of cingulotomy in treating refractory OCD symptoms, and recent work in our and other laboratories investigating ACC-based performance monitoring in this illness.

Reports of OCD comorbidity with neurological disorders such as postencephalitic parkinsonism, Sydenham's chorea, and Tourette's syndrome, as well as with lesions of basal ganglia and/or frontal structures (globus pallidus, caudate nucleus, putamen, ACC, orbitofrontal cortex), have argued for a role for the frontal cortical-striatal circuits in the pathophysiology of OCD. The development of brain-imaging techniques has allowed researchers to explore in vivo the brain pathology potentially underlying OCD symptoms. Generally, these studies—most of them using PET or SPECT (Adams et al. 1993; Baxter et al. 1987; Machlin et al. 1991; Swedo et al. 1989)—confirm strong correlation between the presence of OCD symptoms and abnormalities in function of circuits of the orbital frontal cortex, caudate nucleus, ACC, and thalamus. Most studies have reported increased activity in this circuitry, with further increases associated with symptom provocation. Relatively little emphasis has been given to the role of the ACC in these studies. Most often, activity in this region has been attributed to increased anxiety in OCD patients.

Our model of modularity of medial and lateral frontal cortex contributions to executive control suggests instead that the increased activity in the ACC observed in functional imaging studies might, rather than reflecting an epiphenomenon, be directly associated with important aspects of the symptomatology of OCD. Over a decade ago Pitman (1987) proposed a cybernetic model of OCD in which exaggerated activity in a brain system involved in detecting and correcting errors leads to repetitive signals that actions and mental operations have not been completed satisfactorily, with subsequent obsessional and compulsive behaviors. A number of studies examining the performance of OCD patients on a range of cognitive tasks have suggested that patients' appraisal of their own performance is negatively biased despite their performing in the normal or even superior range (Brown et al. 1994; Constans et al. 1995; McNally and Kohlbeck 1993). Using ERP, Gehring et al. (2000) reported that OCD patients showed an increased ERN compared with control subjects. This was interpreted as reflecting increased error detection in OCD. If our hypothesis is correct and the ACC monitors conflict rather than errors per se, and if the ACC-based performance-monitoring function is enhanced in OCD, then patients should show not only increased error-related activity but also increased activity during correct responses when the task elicits response conflict. Using event-related fMRI, we recently confirmed both predictions. OCD patients showed increased error-related and conflict-related activity in the ACC, and this activity correlated with patients' self-ratings of the severity of their compulsions (Ursu et al. 2000). These results suggest a specific role for hyperactivity of the ACC in the symptomatology of OCD: patients' ACCs provide them with a faulty appraisal of their own functioning and an inappropriate sense that corrective actions need to be taken during what is actually normal task performance.

Conclusions

Within a cognitive-neuroscience–based framework provided by a model of executive functions in which distinct, complementary functions are assigned to dorsolateral and medial regions of frontal cortex, we have described schizophrenia and OCD as disorders of undercontrol and overcontrol, respectively. Schizophrenia, with its prominent disorganization, is likely to be associated with disturbances of the top-down control of attention and working memory associated with the DLPFC and of the performance-monitoring function of the ACC, a double hit to executive functions. Compulsions in OCD may be understood, at least in part, as associated with overactivity of the performance-monitoring function of the ACC, leading to a persistent sense of impaired performance when in fact there is none. These insights are preliminary, and much work remains to be done before a detailed understanding of the neural basis of altered executive functions in these two forms of psychopathology is complete. Our model is incomplete, with only theoretical inferences at this point regarding important such details as the neural coupling of ACC-based performance monitoring with DLPFC-based adjustments in control. However, we believe that these ideas illustrate the potential of the tools and constructs of cognitive neuroscience for shedding light on the mechanisms underlying some of the most disabling aspects of common mental disorders. These tools and constructs may not only provide us with an understanding of the neural basis of clinical symptoms and the mechanism of action of treatments but may ultimately have application in clinical psychiatry, the facilitation of diagnosis, the predicting and tracking of treatment response, and the refining of treatment planning. Cognitive neuroscience will also have important applications in clinical genetics. With the mapping of the human genome and the identification of common genetic polymorphisms, cognitive neuroscientific methods can provide us with neural systems-level phenotypes that are potentially more sensitive, specific correlates of disease-related genetic variation than those identified by phenomenology alone. This approach is referred to as *cognitive neurogenetics* and important initial results related to cognitive dysfunction in schizophrenia are described by Callicott in this volume (see Chapter 1). It is likely that cognitive neuroscience will increasingly become a major focus of clinical neuroscience in the years to come, enhancing our ability to define and investigate many of the most disabling and currently treatment-refractory aspects of the major mental disorders. It is also to be hoped that further developments in cognitive-neuroscience–based functional imaging will eventually inform clinical practice by improving our ability to make a specific diagnosis early in the course of an illness and to predict and track the response to treatment of brain circuitry underlying impaired cognition in the common mental disorders.

References

Adams BL, Warneke LB, McEwan AJ, et al: Single photon emission computerized tomography in obsessive compulsive disorder: a preliminary study. J Psychiatry Neurosci 18(3):109–112, 1993

Andreasen NC, Rezai K, Alliger R, et al: Hypofrontality in neuroleptic naive patients and in patients with chronic schizophrenia: assessment with xenon 133 single photon emission computed tomography and the Tower of London. Arch Gen Psychiatry 49:943–958, 1992

Barch DM, Berenbaum H: Language production and thought disorder in schizophrenia. J Abnorm Psychol 105:81–88, 1996

Barch DM, Carter CS, Usher M, et al: The benefits of distractibility: mechanisms underlying increased Stroop effects in schizophrenia. Schizophr Bull 24(4):749–762, 1999

Barch DM, Carter CS, Braver TS, et al: Selective deficits in prefrontal cortex function in medication naive patients with schizophrenia. Arch Gen Psychiatry (in press)

Baxter LR Jr: Brain imaging as a tool in establishing a theory of brain pathology in obsessive compulsive disorder. J Clin Psychiatry 51(suppl):22–25, 1990

Baxter LR Jr, Phelps ME, Mazziotta JC, et al: Local cerebral glucose metabolic rates in obsessive-compulsive disorder: a comparison with rates in unipolar depression and in normal controls. Arch Gen Psychiatry 44(3):211–218, 1987

Bleuler E: Dementia Praecox or The Group of Schizophrenias (1911). Translated by Zinkin J. New York, International Universities Press, 1950

Botvinick MM, Nystrom L, Fissell K, et al: Conflict monitoring versus selection for action in anterior cingulate cortex. Nature 402(6758): 179–181, 1999

Braff, D: Information processing and attention dysfunction in schizophrenia. Schizophr Bull 19:233–259, 1993

Brown HD, Kosslyn SM, Breiter HC, et al: Can patients with obsessive-compulsive disorder discriminate between percepts and mental images? A signal detection analysis. J Abnorm Psychol 103(3):445–454, 1994

Buchsbaum M: The frontal lobes, basal ganglia and temporal lobes as sites for schizophrenia. Schizophr Bull 16:379–389, 1990

Calloway E, Naghdi S: An information processing model for schizophrenia. Arch Gen Psychiatry 39:339–347, 1982

Carter CS, Robertson LC, Nordahl TE: Abnormal processing of irrelevant information in chronic schizophrenia: selective enhancement of Stroop facilitation. Psychiatry Res 41:137–146, 1992

Carter CS, Robertson LC, Nordahl TE, et al: Spatial working memory deficits and their relationship to negative symptoms in unmedicated schizophrenic patients. Biol Psychiatry 40:930–932, 1996

Carter CS, Mintun M, Nichols T, et al: Anterior cingulate gyrus dysfunction and selective attention dysfunction in schizophrenia: an ^{15}O-H_2O PET study during Stroop task performance. Am J Psychiatry 154:1670–1675, 1997

Carter CS, Braver TS, Barch DM, et al: Anterior cingulate cortex, error detection, and the on line monitoring of performance. Science 280(5364):747–749, 1998

Carter CS, Botvinick MM, Cohen JD: The role of the anterior cingulate cortex in executive processes of cognition. Rev Neurosci 10:49–57, 1999

Carter CS, MacDonald AM, Ross LL, et al: Parsing executive processes: strategic versus evaluative functions of the anterior cingulate cortex. Proc Natl Acad Sci U S A 97:1944–1948, 2000

Clare L, McKenna PJ, Mortimer AM, et al: Memory in schizophrenia: what is impaired and what is preserved. Neuropsychologia 31:1225–1241, 1993

Cohen JD, Servan-Schreiber D: A theory of dopamine function and its role in cognitive deficits in schizophrenia. Schizophr Bull 19(1):85–104, 1993

Cohen JD, Barch DM, Carter CS, et al: Schizophrenic deficits in the processing of context: converging evidence from three theoretically motivated cognitive tasks. J Abnorm Psychology 108:120–133, 1999

Condray R, van Kammen DP, Steinhauer SR, et al: Language comprehension in schizophrenia: trait or state indicator? Biol Psychiatry (A3S) 1:38(5):287–296, 1995

Constans JI, Foa EB, Franklin ME, et al: Memory for actual and imagined events in OC checkers. Behavioral Research and Therapy 33(6):665–671, 1995

Cornblatt BA, Lenzenweger MF, Erlenmeyer-Kimling L: The continuous performance test, identical pairs version, II: contrasting attentional profiles in schizophrenic and depressed patients. J Psychiatric Res 29:65, 1989

Dehaene S, Posner MI, Tucker DM: Localization of a neural system for error detection and compensation. Psychological Science 5(5):303–305, 1994

D'Esposito M, Detre JA, Alsop DC, et al: The neural basis of the central executive system of working memory. Nature 378(6554):279–281, 1995

Docherty NM, Schnur M, Harvey PD: Reference performance and positive and negative thought disorder: a follow-up study of manics and schizophrenics. J Abnorm Psychology 97:437–442, 1988

Docherty NM, DeRosa M, Andreasen, NC: Communication disturbances in schizophrenia and mania. Arch Gen Psychiatry 53:358–364, 1996

Dolan RJ, Fletcher P, Frith CD, et al: Dopaminergic modulation of impaired cognitive activation in the anterior cingulate cortex in schizophrenia. Nature 378(6553):180–182, 1995

Dum RP, Strick PL: Cingulate motor areas, in Neurobiology of Cingulate Cortex and Motor Thalamus. Edited by Vogt B, Gabriel M. Boston, Birkhauser, 1993, pp 415–444

Falkenstein M, Hohnsbein J, Hoorman J, et al: Effects of crossmodal divided attention on late ERP components, II: error processing in choice reaction tasks. Electroencephalogr Clin Neurophysiol 78:447–455, 1991

Feinberg I: Efference copy and corollary discharge: implications for thinking and its disorders. Schizophr Bull 4:636–640, 1978

Frith CD, Done DJ: Experiences of alien control in schizophrenia reflect a disorder in the central monitoring of action. Psychol Med 19:359–363, 1989

Fuster J: The prefrontal cortex: anatomy, physiology and neuropsychology of the frontal lobe. New York, Raven, 1988

Ganguli R, Carter CS, Mintun M, et al: Abnormal cortical physiology in schizophrenia: a PET blood flow study during rest and supraspan memory performance. Biol Psychiatry 4:33–62, 1997

Gazzaniga AM, Lury RB, Mangun GR: Cognitive Neuroscience. New York, Norton and Company, 1998

Gehring WJ, Knight RT: Prefrontal-cingulate interactions in action monitoring. Nat Neurosci 3(5):516–520, 2000

Gehring WJ, Goss B, Coles MGH, et al: A neural system for error detection and compensation. Psychological Science 4(6):385–390, 1993

Gehring WJ, Himle J, Nisenson, LG: Action-monitoring dysfunction in obsessive-compulsive disorder. Psychological Science 11:1–6, 2000

Gold JM, Carpenter C, Randolph C, et al: Auditory working memory and Wisconsin card sorting test performance in patients with schizophrenia. Arch Gen Psychiatry 54(2):159–165, 1997

Goldberg TE, Greenberg RD, Griffin SJ, et al: The effect of Clozapine on cognition and psychiatric symptoms in patients with schizophrenia. Br J Psychiatry 162:43–48, 1993

Goldman-Rakic PS: Circuitry of primate prefrontal cortex and regulation of behavior by representational memory, in Handbook of Physiology: The Nervous System, Vol 5. Bethesda, MD, American Physiological Society, 1987, pp 373–417

Goldman-Rakic PS: Prefrontal cortical dysfunction in schizophrenia: the relevance of working memory, in Psychopathology and the Brain. Edited by Carroll BJ, Barrett JE. New York, Raven, 1991, pp 1–23

Gray J, Feldon J, Rawlins J, et al: The neuropsychology of schizophrenia. Behav Brain Sci 14:1–84, 1990

Green MF: What are the functional consequences of neurocognitive deficits in schizophrenia? Am J Psychiatry 153:321–330, 1996

Green MF: Schizophrenia from a Neurocognitive Perspective: Probing the Impenetrable Darkness. Boston, Allyn & Bacon, 1998

Gur RC, Gur RE: Hypofrontality in schizophrenia: RIP. Lancet 345: 1383–1340, 1995

Hadnezar MM, Buchsbaum MS, Luu C, et al: Decreased anterior cingulate gyrus metabolic rate in schizophrenia. Am J Psychiatry 1564(5): 682–684, 1997

Harvey PD: Speech competence in manic and schizophrenic psychoses: the association between clinically rated thought disorder and comprehension and reference performance. J Abnorm Psychol 92:368–377, 1983

Ingvar DH, Franzen G: Abnormalities of cerebral blood flow distribution in patients with chronic Schizophrenia. Acta Psychiatr Scand 50:425–462, 1974

Keefe RSE, Roitman SEL, Harvey PD, et al: A pen-and-paper human analogue of a monkey prefrontal cortex activation task: spatial working memory in patients with schizophrenia. Schizophr Res 17:25–33, 1995

Kopp B, Rist F: An event-related brain potential substrate of disturbed response monitoring in paranoid schizophrenic patients. J Abnorm Psychol 108:337–346, 1999

Kraepelin E: Dementia Praecox and Paraphrenia (1912). Translated by Barclay RM. Edinburgh, E. & S. Livingstone, 1971

Liddle PF: The psychomotor disorder: disorders of the supervisory mental processes. Behav Neurosci 6:5–14, 1993

Liddle PF, Morris DL: Schizophrenic syndromes and frontal lobe performance. Br J Psychiatry 158:340–345, 1991

Liddle PF, Friston KJ, Frith CD, et al: Patterns of cerebral blood flow in schizophrenia. Br J Psychiatry 160:179–186, 1992

MacDonald AW, Cohen JD, Stenger VA, et al: Dissociating the role of dorsolateral prefrontal and anterior cingulate cortex in cognitive control. Science 288:1835–1838, 2000

Machlin SR, Harris GJ, Pearlson GD, et al: Elevated medial-frontal cerebral blood flow in obsessive-compulsive patients: a SPECT study. Am J Psychiatry 148(9):1240–1242, 1991

Malenka RC, Angel RW, Hampton B, et al: Impaired central error-correcting behavior in schizophrenia. Arch Gen Psychiatry 39:101–107, 1982

Mathalon D, Fedor M, Faustman WO, et al: Self-monitoring abnormalities in schizophrenia: an event-related brain potential study. Proceedings of the Cognitive Neuroscience Society Annual Meeting, San Francisco, CA, 2000, pp 111

McClelland JL, Rumelhart DE: Parallel Distributed Processing. Explorations in the Microstructure of Cognition. Volume 1: Foundations. Cambridge, MA, MIT Press, 1986

McNally RJ, Kohlbeck PA: Reality monitoring in obsessive-compulsive disorder. Beh Res Ther 31:(3), 249–253, 1993

Mesulam MM: A cortical network for directed attention and unilateral neglect. Ann Neurol 10:309–325, 1981

Mirsky AF: Neuropsychological bases of schizophrenia. Annu Rev Psychol 20:321–348, 1969

Morecraft RJ, Louie JL, Shroeder CM, et al: Segregated parallel inputs to the brachial spinal cord from the cingulate motor cortex in the monkey. Neuroreport 8:3933–3938, 1997

Morice R, McNichol D: The comprehension and production of complex syntax in schizophrenia. Cortex 21(4):567–580, 1985

Nuechterlein KH, Dawson ME: Information processing and attentional functioning in the developmental course of schizophrenia disorders. Schizophr Bull 10:160–203, 1984

Pakkenberg B: Pronounced reduction of total neuron number in mediodorsal thalamic nucleus and nucleus accumbens in schizophrenics. Arch Gen Psychiatry 47:1023–1028, 1990

Pardo JV, Fox P, Raichle ME: Localization of a system for sustained attention by positron emission tomography. Nature 349:61–64, 1991

Park S, Holtzman PS: Schizophrenics show spatial working memory deficits. Arch Gen Psychiatry 49:975–982, 1992

Pitman RK: A cybernetic model of obsessive-compulsive psychopathology. Compr Psychiatry 28(4):334–343, 1987

Posner MI, Abdullaev YG: What to image? Anatomy, circuitry and plasticity of human brain function, in Brain Mapping: The Methods. Edited by Toga AW, Mazziota JC. New York, Academic Press, 1996, pp 408–419

Posner MI, Petersen SE: The attention system of the human brain. Annu Rev Neurosci 13:25–42, 1990

Rosvold KE, Mirsky AF, Sarason I, et al: A continuous performance test of brain damage. J Consult Clin Psychol 20:343–350, 1956

Saykin AJ, Gur RC, Gur RE, et al: Neuropsychological function in schizophrenia: selective impairment in memory and learning. Arch Gen Psychiatry 48:618–624, 1991

Schwartz BL, Rosse RB, Deutsch SI: Towards a neuropsychology of memory in schizophrenia Psychopharmacol Bull 28:341–351, 1992

Segalowitz S: Proceedings of the 10th Annual Conference of the Rotman Research Institute, The Frontal Lobes, Toronto, Ontario, Canada, 2000

Shakow D: Segmental set: A theory of the formal psychological deficit in schizophrenia. Arch Gen Psychiatry 6:1–17, 1962

Siegel BV, Buchsbaum MS, Bunney WE, et al: Cortical-striatal-thalamic circuits and brain glucose metabolic activity in 70 unmedicated male schizophrenic patients. Am J Psychiatry 150:1325–1336, 1993

Smith EE, Jonides J: Storage and executive processes in the frontal lobes. Science 283(5408):1657–1661, 1999

Swedo SE, Schapiro MB, Grady CL, et al: Cerebral glucose metabolism in childhood-onset obsessive-compulsive disorder. Arch Gen Psychiatry 46(6):518–523, 1989

Tamlyn D, McKenna P, Mortimer A, et al: Memory impairment in schizophrenia: its extent, affiliations and neuropsychological character. Psychol Med 22:101–115, 1992

Tamminga CA, Thaker GK, Buchanan R, et al: Limbic system abnormalities identified in schizophrenia with fluorodeoxyglucose and neocortical alterations with the deficit syndrome. Arch Gen Psychiatry 49:522–530, 1992

Taylor SF: Cerebral blood flow activation and functional lesions in schizophrenia. Schizophr Res 19(2–3):129–140, 1996

Ursu S, Shear MK, Stenger VA, et al: Functional MRI study of forebrain activation in OCD. Biol Psychiatry, 2000

Weinberger DR, Gallhofer B: Cognitive dysfunction in schizophrenia. Int Clin Psychopharmacol 12(suppl 4):S29–S36, 1997

Weinberger DR, Berman K, Zec R: Physiological dysfunction of dorsolateral prefrontal cortex in schizophrenia, I: regional cerebral blood-flow evidence. Arch Gen Psychiatry 43:114–124, 1986

Young KA, Manaye KF, Liang C, et al: Reduced number of mediodorsal and anterior thalamic neurons in schizophrenia. Biol Psychiatry 47:944–953, 2000

Chapter 3

Functional Magnetic Resonance Imaging in Children and Adolescents

Implications for Research on Emotion

Daniel S. Pine, M.D.

In this chapter the term *emotion* refers to a family of brain states associated with the perception of rewards or punishments; the terms *reward* and *punishment* refer, respectively, to stimuli that an organism will expend effort to obtain or avoid (Rolls 1999). Difficulties with the regulation of emotion represent a basic aspect of many psychiatric disorders (Davidson et al. 2000). Such difficulties often arise early in life and persist into adulthood (Caspi et al. 1996). The purpose of this chapter is to provide a perspective on emotion that integrates neuroscience, clinical psychiatry, and developmental psychology.

This integrative perspective emphasizes the potentially key role of functional magnetic resonance imaging (fMRI) studies in refining pathophysiologic models of pediatric mental disorders. Functional MRI is uniquely suited to such work because it provides a safe and well-tolerated means for noninvasively monitoring associations between brain activity and a range of clinical parameters. Moreover, relative to other noninvasive neuroimaging modalities, fMRI combines excellent spatial resolution for both cortical and subcortical structures with temporal resolution

This research was supported by an NIMH Scientist Development Award for Clinicians to Dr. Daniel S. Pine (K20-MH-01391).

for events occurring on the order of seconds. These are invaluable features for any tool designed to explore neural correlates of emotion. Nevertheless, as of this writing relatively few fMRI studies have examined any aspect of development, let alone specific aspects of emotional development. The proper implementation of such studies will benefit from a clear exposition of key questions that may be answered with this technique. This chapter outlines questions on the pathophysiology of pediatric mood and anxiety disorders that are amenable to study with fMRI. In outlining such questions, I focus on four specific disorders: major depression, generalized anxiety disorder, separation anxiety disorder, and social phobia. Prior studies in epidemiology, family genetics, and neuropsychology suggest that these conditions are distinct from other mood and anxiety disorders, such as obsessive-compulsive disorder (OCD), posttraumatic stress disorder (PTSD), and bipolar disorder (DeBellis et al. 1999; Pine et al. 1998; Rosenberg et al. 1997).

Key questions on pediatric mood and anxiety disorders emerge from a broader developmental perspective on mental illness. Efforts to integrate research in development, clinical psychiatry, and neuroscience follow from recent refinements in models of many mental illnesses other than mood and anxiety disorders. In fact, these refinements show interesting parallels with perspectives on other medical conditions. Early in the course of chronic diseases such as hypertension or dementia, the distinctions between health and illness can remain subtler than the distinctions observable during acute infectious states. In the face of such subtle distinctions, researchers attempting to prevent many chronic illnesses recognize the salience of a developmental perspective, since pathophysiologic processes that culminate in overt illnesses often begin during childhood. Conditions like hypertension (Ewart and Kolodner 1994) and Alzheimer's disease (Snowdon et al. 1996) may be conceptualized as relatively late-stage end products of more basic developmental processes, such as refinements in autonomic regulation or elaboration of basic neurocognitive function. Understanding the unfolding of these developmental processes may provide key insights into pathophysiology.

Research reviewed in this chapter provides an analogous theoretical perspective for adult mood and anxiety disorders. These disorders also can be conceptualized as developmental conditions, and fMRI may ultimately provide the means for directly assessing during childhood and adolescence processes that culminate in chronic mood and anxiety disorders encountered among adults. The first section of this chapter briefly summarizes data supporting such a developmental perspective on the pathophysiology of mood and anxiety disorders. The second reviews data from psychophysiology and neuropsychology that generate hypotheses on neural circuits implicated in mood and anxiety disorders among children as well as adults. In the final section, the relevance of these data for future fMRI studies is delineated.

Developmental Psychopathology Perspectives Applied to Mood and Anxiety Disorders

The school of developmental psychopathology emphasizes the importance of studying changes in symptom patterns across the life span. Research in this area implicitly assumes that pathophysiologic models of many mental illnesses manifesting in adulthood may be refined through research on childhood precursors for the adult condition. The credibility of this perspective derives from two widely replicated findings pertaining to the course and familial nature of mental disorders.

In terms of life course, many chronic mental disorders of adults have roots in childhood. Robins (1978) initially described one developmental aspect of behavior disorders, manifest as a strong relationship between childhood conduct disorder and adult antisocial personality disorder; McGlashan and Hoffman (2000) summarized analogous developmental views of schizophrenia. Developmental perspectives also apply to mood and anxiety disorders. Conditions that typically show adult onset, such as panic disorder and major depression, often develop in the wake of childhood or adolescent mood and anxiety symptoms (Pine et al. 1998, 1999a; Weissman et al. 1997). Similarly, for disorders such as social phobia, children can exhibit symptom profiles that closely parallel the adult syndrome (Pine et al. 1998; Schwartz et al. 1999). However, for the full range of mood and anxiety disorders the proportion of children demonstrating prodromal symptoms or risk factors for an adult disorder is considerably larger than the proportion who ultimately manifest one or another disorder as adults. As a result, the majority of adults with a mood or anxiety disorder will have manifested initial signs of their disorder as children or adolescents, but the majority of children who manifest such initial signs will not ultimately develop full-blown mood or anxiety disorders as adults (Klein and Pine, in press).

These longitudinal data establish an agenda for ongoing research. For example, as reflected in these data, clinicians, patients, and researchers typically encounter difficulty when attempting to precisely date the onset of many conditions. Hence, one goal of current research is to chart changes in symptom profiles across development as they may eventually culminate in adult-type symptom patterns. Similarly, childhood precursors for many adult disorders have been broadly delineated, but the precise nature of associations between child and adult disorders remains poorly understood. For example, some childhood fears may be risk factors for both mood and anxiety disorders during adulthood (Biederman et al. 1995; Weissman et al. 1997); other childhood fears may carry risks for only a particular disorder (Pine et al. 1998); and still other fears may carry no risk for adult mood and anxiety disorders (Feehan et al. 1993). Hence, a second goal of current research is to identify factors that distinguish between children with symptoms who face particularly high or low risks for one adult disorder or another. Data on associations between symptom profiles and brain states, which can be generated using fMRI, may facilitate this second goal. Specifically, from a clinical perspective, refinements in fMRI may help identify impaired children facing a particularly high risk of persistent symptoms.

In terms of familial distribution, equally compelling data emphasize the need for a developmental perspective. The overwhelming majority of mental illnesses show some degree of familial distribution, though there is considerable variability across distinct conditions. Moreover, particularly strong degrees of familial aggregation may occur in early-onset subtypes of mood or anxiety disorders (Goldstein et al. 1994; Weissman et al. 1997). Consistent with longitudinal data on the gradual onset of many adult disorders, children born to parents with many forms of mental illness can manifest relatively subtle signs of an underlying diathesis for the adult condition. For example, children at risk for schizophrenia may show subtle signs of cognitive abnormalities implicated in psychotic disorders (McGlashan and Hoffman 2000), while children at risk for panic disorder may show subtle signs of deficient regulation in fear-related behaviors (Merikangas et al. 1999).

As in the area of life-course research, these results establish the need for a perspective that integrates research on development, psychopathology, and neuroscience. For example, while familial distribution of many illnesses is well-established, limited insights exist on mechanisms through which conditions are transmitted from parents to children. Mechanistic understanding requires delineation of the underlying genetic and neural substrate from which disorders develop, carrying potential major implications for early identification of at-risk children. Similarly, to facilitate effective prevention and early intervention, research must delineate the manner in which this underlying substrate changes with development to ultimately produce overtly manifest symptoms. As in the area of longitudinal course, advances in fMRI may provide a clinical tool for predicting risk. Mechanisms associated with parent-child transmission of mental illnesses might eventually be visualized with fMRI. These methods might be used to identify high-risk children in particular need of intervention.

Taken together, longitudinal and family studies outline broad associations between mental disorders in children and adults. Nevertheless, such studies do not suffice for the detailed conceptualization of particular disorders or of the pathophysiologic processes that connect child and adult disorders. As articulated by Frith (1991) and illustrated in Figure 3–1, a hierarchical perspective provides a novel view of such questions. In this perspective, constructs related to mental illnesses extend from overt symp-

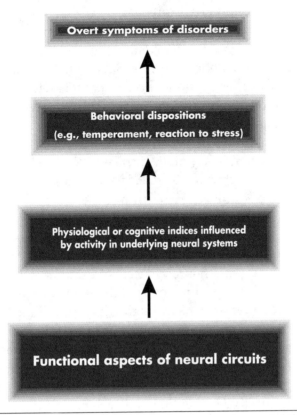

Figure 3–1. Hierarchical model of phenomena in mental illness.

toms of disorders to the underlying neural substrata. From the perspective of current nosology, symptomatic manifestations of some distinct childhood mental disorders (e.g., social phobia) exhibit close parallels with symptomatic manifestations of similarly defined adult disorders (Pine et al. 1998; Schwartz et al. 1999). A disorder in children, such as separation anxiety disorder, may also relate to a nosologically distinct adult disorder such as panic disorder (Capps et al. 1996; Klein and Pine, in press; Weissman et al. 1997). At a slightly deeper conceptual level, symptoms of disorders specified in DSM-IV (American Psychiatric Association 1994) may arise from broad behavioral dispositional tendencies not fully captured in DSM-IV. Such dispositional tendencies might be captured in measures of temperamental constructs, such as behavioral inhibition or avoidant behavioral styles, which can show relatively broad associations with a range of mental syndromes (Biederman et al. 1995). Alternatively, such tendencies might be captured in ratings of children's characteristic reactions to motivational stimuli or standardized stressors, as assessed using self-ratings and observational measures.

At a still deeper level, behavioral dispositional tendencies are thought to reflect functional aspects of neural systems involved in the regulation of behaviors and emotional states. Dispositional tendencies, like other integrative aspects of the nervous system, are thought to be modularized in the brain, regulated by a network of interconnected brain regions. Activity in these networks can be indirectly inferred through physiologic or cognitive measures; regulation capacities in underlying brain systems are reflected in physiologic, neurohormonal, and cognitive profiles. For example, Kagan's construct of behavioral inhibition relates to activity in fear circuits, assessed through inferential physiologic measures (Kagan 1995). Similarly, risk for anxiety associated with functional aspects of relevant brain circuits may be reflected in a heightened attentional bias for threat cues (Mathews and Mac-Loed 1994; McNally 1996, 1997) or abnormalities in startle regulation (Merikangas et al. 1999). Finally, advances in brain imaging enable direct assessment of the underlying substrate from which mental disorders arise, and fMRI provides perhaps the best available avenue for such assessments in children.

Ultimately, fMRI studies may be used to define the neural substrate of mood and anxiety disorders. However, given the complexity of the pathophysiologic processes, such efforts will benefit from research that establishes ties between neural processes and functional aspects of neural systems as reflected in physiologic or cognitive indices.

Data Implicating Neural Circuits in Pediatric Mood and Anxiety Disorders

Cognitive and physiological data implicate common brain regions in aspects of emotion regulation among humans and animals. These data generate questions that are amenable to systematic study with fMRI. In particular, neuroscience research on processes involved in response to punishments and rewards generates insights on the pathophysiology of mood and anxiety disorders. These basic processes affect attention and memory, cognitive processes perturbed in mood and anxiety disorders. Each process is tractable in fMRI experiments among children and adolescents, based on the wealth of available data among adults.

Response to Danger

Considerable enthusiasm for neuroscientific study of emotion follows from research on fear conditioning (Davis 1998; LeDoux 1996, 1998). Fear conditioning refers to the process through which organisms learn to associate formerly neutral stimuli with potentially dangerous or punishing stimuli. In the classic fear conditioning experiment, a neutral stimulus, such as a tone or a light, is paired with an aversive stimulus, such as a shock, air puff, or loud noise. The formerly neutral conditioned stimulus comes to elicit behavior and physiologic responses typical for the innately aversive unconditioned stimulus. The organism also develops a fear-related response to the chamber in which the experiment was implemented, a process known as *contextual conditioning*.

Enthusiasm for research on these processes in humans derives from the mechanistic understanding of associated neural processes. Brain circuits that regulate fear conditioning have been delineated down to the molecular level (Crestani et al. 1999; Squire and Kandel 1999). While these circuits involve an array of brain structures, components of the amygdala are centrally involved. Enthusiasm for applications of fear conditioning research to human disorders derives from parallels between aspects of fear conditioning across mammalian species and clinical fear states in humans. Both fear conditioning in animals and clinical fear states in humans are characterized by avoidance behavior and by parallel changes in vigilance and autonomic regulation. Both processes involve a decrease in hedonic activity. Moreover, experimental lesions abolish fear conditioning in animals, and amygdala lesions in humans interfere with fear conditioning as well as with a range of related processes (Davis 1998; LeDoux 1996, 1998). Despite these parallels, fear conditioning as classically studied in the rodent provides only indirect insights into the pathophysiology of anxiety disorders. Classically defined cue-specific fear conditioning appears normal in many anxiety disorders (Klein and Pine, in press). Conversely, in research with rodents, fear conditioning remains unaffected by pharmacological agents that effectively treat anxiety disorders (Cassella and Davis 1985).

Such inconsistencies between clinical fear states and fear conditioning have been attributed to at least two underlying processes. First, such differences may be understandable through hierarchical perspectives. For example, fear conditioning may relate more strongly to risk for anxiety or broad dispositional tendencies, as opposed to clinical disorders. Consistent with this possibility, children at risk for anxiety disorders, by virtue of temperament or parental histories, show some signs of enhanced fear conditioning, though not all studies note such findings (Kagan 1995; Merikangas et al. 1999). Second, some process associated *with* fear conditioning may relate more closely to anxiety disorders than does fear conditioning per se. For example, healthy organisms proficiently differentiate dangerous stimuli or situations from similar-appearing but harmless situations; anxiety disorders may result from a failure to make such distinctions (Crestani et al. 1999). Such differentiations may become particularly difficult across contexts, for example, when attempting to determine danger associated with a scream in a movie theater as opposed to a scream in a dark alley. Alternatively, clinical anxiety disorders may result more from processes associated with responses to unconditioned stimuli, as opposed to the pairing of conditioned and unconditioned stimuli. Patients with various anxiety disorders show enhanced reactivity upon entering laboratory situations. This may reflect differences in processes associated with novelty perception or the anticipation of potentially aversive events.

Consistent with this second conceptualization, Davis (1998) provides a compelling integration of research on fear conditioning and clinical psychopathology. Normal, adaptive fear (in this conceptualization) is modeled by the classic fear conditioning experiment. Anxiety disorders are modeled by either contextually elicited or innate fears, phenomena that Davis (1998) labels *anxiety.* Fear in rodents of a well-lit open field or fear in humans of a dark room provides an example of such contextual, innate forms of anxiety.

Response to Reward

Research on neural correlates of reward-related behaviors is a second area of neuroscience relevant to pathophysiologic models of pediatric mood and anxiety disorders. Through research on intracranial self-stimulation, a neural network has been delineated that mediates perception and response to rewards (Rolls 1999). This network encompasses monoamine systems ascending from the brainstem and regions that are heavily innervated by these systems, including the basal ganglia and forebrain, particularly components of the frontal cortex. The dopamine system plays a particularly important role in reward-related behavior, as does the nucleus accumbens in the basal ganglia and the ventral prefrontal region in the cortex (Rolls 1999). Animals will expend effort to receive direct stimulation to a network encompassing these brain regions or to obtain compounds, such as amphetamines, that activate these brain regions. Similarly, components of the ventral prefrontal cortex play a prominent role in flexible representation of stimuli's motivational properties (Rolls 1999). The ventral prefrontal cortex may become particularly engaged when the rewarding properties of stimuli change, as in stimulus reversal paradigms. Parenthetically, such functional aspects of the ventral prefrontal cortex may be reflected in some fear-related processes, such as habituation (LeDoux 1996). Ventral prefrontal lesions interfere with this process, which involves perceiving changes in associations among neutral and punishing (as opposed to rewarding) stimuli (Rolls 1999).

Psychophysiologic studies implicate aberrant reward-related processes in depression. Depressed adults show a range of psychophysiologic abnormalities during presentations of rewarding stimuli (Davidson et al. 2000). These include abnormal modulation of the startle reflex and aberrant lateralization of neural activity in the frontal lobes, as reflected in electroencephalograms (Davidson 1998; Lang et al. 1998). Such psychophysiologic data show both continuity and discontinuity with data in anxiety disorders. Both anxiety and depression are associated with abnormal responses to various negatively valenced stimuli, whereas depression may also be uniquely associated with abnormal responses to positive stimuli (Allen et al. 1999; Bruder et al. 1999a; Lang et al. 1998). Such data are consistent with theories that group phenomenological aspects of mood and anxiety disorders into three categories: negative affect, response to rewards, and response to danger. Both anxiety and depression are associated with high negative-affect ratings, whereas depression is particularly linked to deficiencies in reward-related processes and anxiety to deficiencies in danger-related processes. As articulated by Davidson (1998) and Bruder et al. (1999a), this categorization may be reflected by two neural gradients running from left to right and anterior to posterior. In anterior brain regions, both patients with anxiety and patients with depression may show enhanced engagement of the right hemisphere, reflecting a tendency to activate brain systems that facilitate withdrawal from danger. In posterior brain regions patients with anxiety and depression may differ, with depressed patients showing more engagement of the left posterior hemisphere (Bruder et al. 1999a, 1999b). Such posterior hemisphere abnormalities also appear in adolescence (Kentgen et al., in press) and may reflect a shutting down of brain systems associated with arousal or orientation.

Depressed adults also show a pattern of cognitive abnormalities indicative of abnormal sensitivity to rewarding stimuli or to the loss of rewards. Such deficits, for example, are manifest on decision-making tasks (Murphy et al. 1999; Rogers et al. 1999), in response to failure (Elliott et al. 1996), or in brain-asymmetry patterns (Bruder et al. 1999b). Similarly, among adolescents this reduced sensitivity to rewards may be reflected in performance on cognitive tasks (e.g., dichotic listening test) that differentially engage the right and left posterior regions (Pine et al. 2000). Such cognitive abnormalities show interesting parallels with subjective aspects of depression. For example, the symptom of anhedonia is an abnormal subjective experience of rewarding stimuli. This symptom appears to be a particularly robust predictor among adolescents of later major depressive episodes (Pine et al. 1999a).

Attention and Memory

Abnormalities in the processing of dangerous or rewarding stimuli affect other psychological processes, particularly attention and memory. These effects are thought to derive from interactions between the brain systems described above with other brain systems devoted to such basic cognitive processes. For attention, brain circuits involved in response to danger are thought to influence activity in frontal, parietal, and temporal regions and in the cingulate gyrus (Carter et al. 2000; Davis 1998; LeDoux 1996; MacDonald et al. 2000; McNally 1996). For memory, the hippocampus and the frontal and temporal cortices may represent key brain regions (Casey et al. 1995; McNally 1997; Mineka and Sutton 1992; Mori et al. 1999; Squire and Kandel 1999).

Regarding danger-related processes and clinical anxiety disorders, the most compelling data document effects of aversive or potentially dangerous stimuli on attention. A state of vigilance represents an essential component of fear states, induced either through conditioning or presentation of unconditioned stimuli. Vigilance involves attentional bias for stimuli associated with potential danger (McNally 1997; Mineka and Sutton 1992; Vasey et al. 1996). In humans, this state can be assessed by comparing reaction times to various stimuli or by examining the disrupting effects of various stimuli on competing cognitive processes (Mathews and MacLoed 1994; Mogg and Bradley 1999; Williams et al. 1996). Much like adults, children with anxiety disorders consistently exhibit enhanced vigilance or bias for threat cues on these tasks (Bradley et al. 1999; Taghavi et al. 1999; Vasey et al. 1996).

For depression, the most compelling data in this area document effects on memory. There is some evidence for overall deficit in memory among depressed adults (Zakzanis et al. 1998). However, recent interest focuses more on interactions between mnemonic and motivational processes. The degree to which stimuli are encoded in memory is affected by the emotional content and arousing nature of the stimulus (Lang et al. 1998; Lundh and Ost 1996; McNally 1997). This influence is manifest as a memory advantage for arousing stimuli. The underlying neural circuitry of this process has been delineated through both lesion studies in animals and brain imaging studies in humans (Cahill 1999;

Phelps and Anderson 1997). Brain circuits involving the amygdala and the hippocampus appear to be centrally involved. Adults with major depression tend to show a greater memory advantage for arousing, negatively valenced stimuli (Mathews and Mac-Loed 1994; Mineka and Sutton 1992). In general, this effect tends to be weaker in anxiety disorders, though some groups of anxious patients may also show abnormal memory bias (McNally 1997).

Relevance of Developmental Psychopathology

Such cognitive data provide insights on brain circuits potentially involved in mood and anxiety disorders. However, the degree to which such cognitive abnormalities represent epiphenomena—as opposed to processes associated with risk or causative abnormalities—remains unclear. For example, because abnormalities in attention or memory can be altered by experience, including effective treatment, they may represent epiphenomena. Because the initial signs of mood and anxiety disorders often emerge during childhood, documenting comparable cognitive correlates of mood or anxiety across the life span or even prior to disorder onset might lend some support to causative theories. In general, cognitive correlates of mood and anxiety disorders in children show parallels with cognitive correlates of mood and anxiety disorders in adults (Pine et al. 1999b, 2000; Taghavi et al. 1999; Vasey et al. 1996). However, such findings may still reflect the influences of problems with mood or anxiety on cognitive processes in children.

Studies of at-risk populations of children and adolescents may lend further support to theories attributing causal roles to underlying cognitive processes in the genesis of mood and anxiety disorders. While relatively limited evidence exists in this area, research on the manner in which puberty influences cognitive and emotional development provides some support. Rates of major depression and select forms of anxiety, such as panic attacks, show marked increases during adolescence. While such increases might be attributable to either age-related or puberty-related processes, recent studies suggest closer associations with puberty (Angold et al. 1998, 1999). Aspects of neural and cognitive development may show parallel associations with puberty. Brain regions implicated in response to danger or rewards mature around puberty (Giedd et al. 1999; Sowell et al. 1999; Thompson et al. 2000), but the degree to which these maturational changes are tied to puberty (as opposed to chronological age) remains unclear. More extensive data link select cognitive processes specifically to puberty (Diamond et al. 1983; Keating 1990; Keating and Sasse 1996). Based on the tie between emotional problems and puberty, neurodevelopmental and cognitive changes associated with puberty may relate to neural systems that facilitate risk for mood and anxiety disorders during adolescence.

Using fMRI to Probe Developmental Dysfunction in Neural Circuits

Because MRI research on pediatric mood and anxiety disorders remains limited, this section briefly summarizes the available data from both structural and functional MRI studies in children and adolescents. Relevant studies in adults are then summarized.

Structural MRI Studies of Pediatric Mood and Anxiety Disorders

For at least two reasons, fMRI studies should be conducted in the context of detailed structural MRI studies on brain morphometry. First, such structural MRI studies remain free of artifacts or biases that can influence fMRI results. As a result, they may enable valid inferences regarding the implication of various brain regions in mental illness. For example, in research on schizophrenia, structural MRI studies delineated brain regions where functional abnormalities frequently have been detected (Wright et al. 2000). Nevertheless, an absence of structural differences does not necessarily exclude a functional abnormality. Particularly in episodic conditions such as mood and anxiety disorders, functional abnormalities may emerge against a backdrop of normal brain structure (Davidson 1998). Second, studies of adults note that structural MRI data can be used to constrain functional neuroimaging data. For example, Drevets et al. (1997) note that volume differences in ventral prefrontal regions can impact on comparisons of brain activity in these regions.

As of this writing, only two studies have compared brain structure in healthy children and adolescents with brain structure in children having one of the mood or anxiety disorders discussed in this chapter. First, consistent with studies implicating the amygdala in fear conditioning, DeBellis et al. (2000) found a larger right amygdala in 10 children with generalized anxiety disorder, as compared to the amygdala in 20 healthy, matched children. This result is reminiscent of Mori et al. (1999), who found that larger amygdala volume predicted better memory for emotional aspects of the 1995 earthquake in Kobe, Japan. Interestingly, these findings contrast to those for OCD, at least among adults, where reduced rather than enlarged amygdala volumes have been reported (Szeszko et al. 1999). Second, consistent with studies of adults implicating the prefrontal cortex in mood regulation, Steingard et al. (1996) found smaller prefrontal volumes in children and adolescents with major depression.

A range of other structural data might inform efforts to conduct future studies in pediatric mood and anxiety disorders. For example, much research has examined brain volumes in disorders that are often comorbid with the mood and anxiety disorders discussed in this chapter. These include attention deficit disorder (Pine et al., in press), PTSD (DeBellis et al. 1999), and OCD (Rosenberg et al. 1997). As a result, effects of such comorbid disorders on brain volumes in mood and anxiety disorders must be considered. Similarly, studies among adults suggest that associations between mood disorders and brain structure may be influenced by the course of the disorder. Hippocampal abnormalities, for example, may appear most likely after chronic or repeated episodes of major depression (Sheline et al. 1996). Finally, studies among adults suggest the importance of considering familial risk when contrasting healthy and ill groups, as healthy relatives of psychiatric patients may also show abnormalities in brain structure (Drevets et al. 1997; Staal et al. 2000).

Functional MRI Studies

Through fMRI, changes in brain activity associated with various events or mental processes can be visualized noninvasively. Perhaps the most frequently employed fMRI method is the *blood oxygen level dependent* (BOLD) technique. With this method, changes in the magnetic resonance (MR) signal result from changes in the ratio of oxy- to deoxyhemoglobin. When a brain region is engaged by a specific cognitive task, MR signal is generally thought to increase as a result of an increase in the oxy- to deoxyhemoglobin ratio. Most fMRI studies require implementation of procedures for isolating specific cognitive functions. Such procedures can rely on comparisons between an experimental and control task that theoretically differ only on this specific cognitive function. Alternatively, event-related methods can link particular events to changes in brain activity. Because most mental operations relevant to psychiatric disorders represent complex phenomena, it is difficult to precisely isolate cognitive functions and their associated changes in BOLD signal.

Thus, no fMRI studies have examined functional aspects of the pediatric mood and anxiety disorders covered in the current chapter. In fact, only a handful of fMRI studies have examined brain circuitry engaged in neurologically intact children by any of the psychological processes reviewed in this chapter (Casey et al. 1995; Nelson et al. 2000; Thomas et al. 1999, 2000). As a result, this chapter reviews data from relevant studies among adults on psychological processes implicated in both pediatric and adult disorders. These include fear-related and reward-related processes as well as attention and memory. A key aspect of implementing such studies among children will be refining procedures for conducting fMRI. For example, in studies of children, the use of fMRI simulators is thought to facilitate research on brain-behavior associations.

Fear-Related Processes

Considerable fMRI data from adults delineate brain regions engaged by both conditioned and unconditioned stimuli. These data show interesting parallels with animal-based work delineating relevant brain circuits. As reviewed by Buchel and Dolan (2000), five fMRI studies have examined brain regions engaged during fear-conditioning experiments. While a series of studies also examine engaged brain regions with positron emission tomography (PET), these studies are not reviewed in the current chapter, given differences in temporal and spatial resolution between PET and fMRI. LaBar et al. (1998) documented right amygdala activation during fear conditioning as well as a correlation between skin conductance and amygdala responses in these subjects. In two studies, Buchel et al. (1999, 2000) also documented amygdala activation during fear conditioning. In the latter study, Buchel and colleagues employed a trace-conditioning paradigm. Studies in rodents implicate the hippocampus in trace conditioning, consistent with the fMRI data for humans given by Buchel et al. (2000). Schneider et al. (1999) documented fear conditioning in patients with social phobia but not in healthy adults, using faces as conditioned stimuli and odors as unconditioned stimuli. Finally, Ploghous et al. (1999) failed to find amygdala activation using heat pain as an unconditioned stimulus, though it is not clear if the field of view for this study covered the medial temporal lobe. These fMRI studies in adults are relevant to studies in pediatric mood and anxiety disorders, given psychophysiological data from Merikangas et al. (1999) implicating fear conditioning in childhood risk for anxiety. Functional MRI studies of fear conditioning in children analogously may delineate functional abnormalities in relevant brain regions that confer risk for later anxiety.

Beyond studies of fear conditioning, other fMRI research among adults explores brain regions engaged by perception of aversive stimuli. This includes research on noxious odors, upsetting visual scenes, and painful stimuli. Across studies, limbic structures are consistently engaged by such stimuli. These findings may be indirectly relevant for mood and anxiety disorders, given hypotheses implicating a generally abnormal response to a range of aversive stimuli in these disorders (Davidson 1998) However, with a few notable exceptions (see Irwin et al. 1996; Lang et al. 1998), stimuli employed in these fMRI studies show only relatively broad similarities with stimuli employed in psychological research with psychiatric patients. Standard emotionally evocative pictures provide one avenue for integrating fMRI and previous psychophysiological studies on emotional processes (Lang et al. 1998).

Research with facial stimuli may provide a particularly important avenue for such integration, given knowledge on developmental, neuroanatomical, and psychopathological aspects of face processing (McClure 2000; Mogg and Bradley 1999). Considerable fMRI research among healthy adults documents engagement of limbic brain regions by facial stimuli (Breiter et al. 1996; Phillips et al. 1998; Whalen et al. 1998). Consistent with data from patients with brain lesions, there is evidence of neuroanatomical specificity in fMRI studies across various emotional facial displays; the amygdala appears particularly sensitive to fearful expressions, the striatum and insula to disgust, and ventral prefrontal regions to anger (Breiter et al. 1996; Phillips et al. 1997; Whalen et al. 1998). Studies have only begun to apply these techniques to psychiatric patients. Birbaumer et al. (1998) documented differential sensitivity of the amygdala to facial expressions in social phobia.

Functional MRI studies documenting consistent engagement of limbic regions by emotionally salient facial expressions provide important insights for research in pediatric mood and anxiety disorders. The amygdala is thought to affect activity in a larger network devoted to perceiving and responding to motivational stimuli (Buchel and Dolan 2000). For example, processing of emotionally salient faces may involve simultaneous recruitment of the amygdala and ventral temporal regions frequently implicated in face processing (Ishai et al. 1999; Kanwisher et al. 1997; Lang et al. 1998). These ventral brain regions are in turn implicated in aspects of brain plasticity, a process that may underlie aspects of cognitive development. Humans are thought to treat stimuli such as faces as particularly salient objects, as evidenced by the unique psychological and psychophysiological responses to such stimuli. Functional MRI studies suggest that such specialized processing tends to develop over time, possibly through changes in the ventral temporal region (Gauthier et al. 1999). As a result, passive viewing of faces may elicit distinct brain activation patterns across development and across developmental psychopathologies. Consistent with this possibility, Thomas et al. (2000) document differences in amygdala activation to emotionally evocative faces among healthy and anxious adolescents and adults.

The wealth of data on face processing may also be used to inform fMRI studies of attentional or mnemonic processes in mood and anxiety disorders. Mogg and Bradley (1999) document vigilance for angry faces in anxiety disorders, while Lundh and Ost (1996) document a memory bias for hostile faces in social phobia. Preliminary studies suggest a role for attentional or mnemonic processes in pediatric anxiety (Merikangas et al. 1999; Pine et al. 1998; Vasey et al. 1996). As a result, differential attention to or memory for emotionally expressive faces in pediatric anxiety might be reflected in brain activation patterns on fMRI as well as behavioral indices of attention and memory.

Response to Reward

As with studies on neural aspects of processing punishing stimuli, existing fMRI studies in adults also examine various aspects of reward-related behaviors. These include both the processing of rewarding stimuli and the role of rewards in decision making.

A series of studies have examined the degree to which various brain regions are engaged by perception of positively valenced stimuli. These have included happy facial expressions, standardized emotionally evocative slides, and financial rewards (Elliott et al. 2000; Lang et al. 1998).

In general, studies in this area document engagement of brain regions implicated in brain reward among lower mammals. Similarly, Teasdale et al. (1999) examined brain regions engaged by stimuli that were affectively neutral but associated with positively valenced stimuli. Emotion was elicited through verbal cues, and cues eliciting positive emotions selectively engaged the medial frontal region, anterior cingulate, caudate nuclei, and precentral gyrus.

Studies also note the engagement of reward-related brain regions when subjects make decisions that impact on reward-related processes. Using PET, Rodgers et al. (1999) observed engagement of the ventral prefrontal cortex during such a decision/reward task. Similarly, using fMRI, Elliott et al. (2000) and Zalla et al. (2000) observed the engagement of reward-related brain regions in tasks that involve guessing and delivery of reward. Such studies implicate the ventral frontal region and other reward-relevant structures in reward processes among humans. These results are reminiscent of studies of brain structure and resting cerebral metabolism in adult major depression (Drevets et al. 1997). In particular, adults with familial forms of major depression exhibit functional and structural abnormalities in the ventral components of the prefrontal cortex (Drevets 1998).

Attention and Memory

Considerable fMRI research among adults establishes brain regions engaged during tasks that affect attention and memory. As reviewed above, behavioral studies document abnormal performance of such tasks among children and adults with mood or anxiety disorders. As a result, the extensive prior fMRI data on neural correlates of attention and memory provide a guide for future studies of pediatric mood and anxiety disorders.

Functional MRI studies implicate separable brain circuits in distinct components of attention (Carter et al. 2000; MacDonald et al. 2000). Such work is relevant to prior research in anxiety disorders. For example, components of the cingulate gyrus have been implicated in aspects of attentional conflict or allocation (Carter et al. 2000). In situations where there are competing demands on attentional systems, the cingulate gyrus may be involved in weighing alternative choices for further processing. During such weighing of alternative choices, individuals at risk for anxiety disorders are hypothesized to display a bias for potentially dangerous stimuli. Such bias may be manifest as abnormal reaction times during conflict tasks, such as the Stroop task, where existing fMRI studies document the engagement of the cingulate gyrus (Peterson et al. 1998; Isenberg et al. 1999). However, the degree to which engagement of this region varies as a function of performance remains unclear. Given performance differences among patient groups, fMRI studies of such attentional processes may enable the mapping of neural circuits involved in risk for anxiety disorders. Nevertheless, interpretation of between-group differences in brain activation patterns is complicated for fMRI tasks (Callicott et al. 1999).

Functional MRI studies have also documented involvement of distinct brain regions in various aspects of memory. For example, prefrontal engagement during declarative (Squire and Kandel 1999) and working memory (Callicott et al. 1998; Casey et al. 1995) tasks has been robustly demonstrated with fMRI, while alterations in cortical activation have been repeatedly demonstrated during priming, an elemental form of memory (Henson and Shallice 1999). Of particular relevance to mood and anxiety disorders is the considerable research that examines the manner in which the emotional content of to-be-remembered material influences recall and brain activation patterns (Blaney 1986). Declarative forms of memory that involve conscious recollection of previously presented material engage a range of brain regions, including areas of the prefrontal cortex, posterior cortex, and medial temporal lobe, particularly the hippocampus. The emotional content or arousing nature of a stimulus influences the degree to which it may be later recalled, with arousing material being more readily recalled than unarousing stimuli (Lang et al. 1998). Prior studies with PET as well as fMRI suggest that this modulatory effect of arousal may derive from amygdala influences on activity in the hippocampal formation (Cahill 1999). During encoding, both amygdala activity and correlations between amygdala and hippocampal activity may predict the degree to which emotional material will be recalled. Abnormalities in such associations between amygdala and hippocampal activity may relate to mnemonic bias in depression.

Development and Plasticity

Given the paucity of available studies, the most appropriate methods for studying developmental processes with fMRI have yet to be defined. In general, activations in fMRI experiments reflect changes in the ratio of oxygenated to deoxygenated hemoglobin. Developmental factors might impact on various aspects of such activations, including the amplitude or the extent of activations. Hypotheses on such changes should be grounded in current theories of brain development, which tend to emphasize the role of changes in connectivity among brain regions (Karmiloff-Smith 1998; Kolb 1999). Such changes produce perturbations in either height or extent of activations.

The regulation of peripheral hemodynamics also changes during development. Since the fMRI signal represents a hemodynamic signal of central origin, changes in central hemodynamics could also potentially influence the fMRI signal. Finally, developmentally oriented fMRI studies should be grounded in the wealth of available behavioral data on cognitive development. However, fMRI studies of adults document complex relationships between task performance and brain activation patterns. Under some circumstances, such as during certain memory encoding exercises, increased brain activation predicts enhanced performance. Nevertheless, under other circumstances, such as during perceptual priming, reduced brain activation predicts enhanced performance. Callicott et al. (1999) suggest that still other cognitive functions show inverted-U–shaped associations with brain activation patterns. Functional MRI studies in children and adolescents further complicate this area by adding development as a factor that may influence associations between activation and performance.

Conclusions

Data from longitudinal and family studies establish the developmental nature of mood and anxiety disorders. However, pathophysiologic theories of these conditions remain relatively poorly specified. Considerable enthusiasm for advances in this area has emerged from a wealth of neuroscience data on brain circuitry that underlies emotion. Functional MRI provides perhaps the best method for integrating clinical developmental insights with neuroscientific perspectives. Due to the difficulty of such work, virtually no fMRI research examines the neural basis of emotional processes in children and adolescents. Studies among adults do outline fMRI procedures for examining emotional processes. Many of these studies examine processes, such as fear conditioning, which data implicate in childhood mood or anxiety disorders. Such studies have set the stage for a wealth of fMRI research on emotional processes in children and adolescents.

References

Allen NB, Trinder J, Brennan C: Affective startle modulation in clinical depression: preliminary findings. Biol Psychiatry 46:542–550, 1999

American Psychiatric Association: Diagnostic and Statistical Manual of Mental Disorders, 4th Edition. Washington, DC, American Psychiatric Association, 1994

Angold A, Costello EJ, Worthman CM: Puberty and depression: the roles of age, pubertal status and pubertal timing. Psychol Med 28:51–61, 1998

Angold A, Costello EJ, Erkanli A, et al: Pubertal changes in hormone levels and depression in girls. Psychol Med 29:1043–1053, 1999

Biederman J, Rosenbaum JF, Chaloff J, et al: Behavioral inhibition as a risk factor for anxiety disorders, in Anxiety Disorders in Children and Adolescents. Edited by March J. New York, Guilford, 1995, pp 61–81

Birbaumer N, Gould W, Diedrich O, et al: fMRI reveals amygdala activation to human faces in social phobics. Neuroreport 9:1223–1226, 1998

Blaney PH: Affect and memory: a review. Psychol Bull 99:229–246, 1986

Bradley BP, Mogg K, White J, et al: Attentional bias for emotional faces in generalized anxiety disorder. Br J Clin Psychol 38:267–278, 1999

Breiter HC, Etcoff JL, Whalen PJ, et al: Response and habituation of the human amygdala during visual processing of facial expression. Neuron 17:875–887, 1996

Bruder GE, Tenke CE, Stewart JW, et al: Predictors of therapeutic response to treatments for depression: a review of electrophysiologic and dichotic listening studies. CNS Spectrums 4, 30–36, 1999a

Bruder, GE, Wexler BE, Stewart JW, et al: Perceptual asymmetry differences between major depression with or without a comorbid anxiety disorder: a dichotic listening study. J Abnorm Psychol 108:233–239, 1999b

Buchel C, Dolan RJ: Classical fear conditioning in functional neuroimaging. Curr Opin Neurobiol 10:219–223, 2000

Buchel C, Morris J, Dolan RJ, et al: Brain systems mediating aversive conditioning: an event-related fMRI study. Neuron 20:937–945, 1998

Buchel C, Dolan RJ, Armony J, et al: Amygdala-hippocampal involvement in human aversive trace conditioning revealed through event related fMRI. J Neurosci 19:10869–10876, 1999

Cahill L: A neurobiological perspective on emotionally influenced, long-term memory. Semin Clin Neuropsychiatry 4:266–273, 1999

Callicott JH, Ramsey NF, Tallent K, et al: Functional magnetic resonance imaging brain mapping in psychiatry: methodological issues illustrated in a study of working memory in schizophrenia. Neuropsychopharmacology 18:186–196, 1998

Callicott JH, Mattay VS, Bertolino A, et al: Physiological characteristics of capacity constraints in working memory as revealed by functional MRI. Cereb Cortex 9:20–26, 1999

Capps L, Sigman M, Sena R, et al: Fear, anxiety and perceived control in children of agoraphobic parents. J Child Psychol Psychiatry 37:445–452, 1996

Carter CS, Macdonald AM, Botvinick M, et al: Parsing executive processes: strategic vs. evaluative functions of the anterior cingulate cortex. Proc Natl Acad Sci U S A 15(97):1944–1949, 2000

Casey BJ, Cohen JD, Jezzard P, et al: Activation of prefrontal cortex in children during a nonspatial working memory task with functional MRI. NeuroImage 2:221–229, 1995

Caspi A, Moffitt TE, Newman DL, et al: Behavioral observations at age 3 years predict adult psychiatric disorders: longitudinal evidence from a birth cohort. Arch Gen Psychiatry 53:1033–1039, 1996

Cassella JV, Davis M. Fear-enhanced acoustic startle is not attenuated by acute or chronic imipramine. Pyschopharmacology 87:278–282, 1985

Crestani F, Lorez M, Baer K, et al: Decreased GABA-receptor clustering results in enhanced anxiety and a bias for threat cues. Nat Neurosci 2:833–839, 1999

Davidson RJ. Anterior electrophysiological asymmetries, emotion, and depression: conceptual and methodological conundrums. Psychophysiology 35:607–614, 1998

Davidson RJ, Putnam KM, Larson CL: Dysfunction in the neural circuitry of emotion regulation: a possible prelude to violence. Science 289:591–594, 2000

Davis M: Are different parts of the amygdala involved in fear versus anxiety? Biol Psychiatry 44:1239–1247, 1998

DeBellis MD, Keshavan MS, Clark DB, et al: A. E. Bennett Research Award: developmental traumatology, II: brain development. Biol Psychiatry 45:1271–1284, 1999

DeBellis MD, Casey BJ, Dahl RE, et al: A pilot study of amygdala volumes in pediatric generalized anxiety disorder. Biol Psychiatry 48:51–57, 2000

Diamond R, Carey S, Back KJ: Genetic influences on the development of spatial skills during early adolescence. Cognition 13:167–185, 1983

Drevets WC: Functional neuroimaging studies of depression: the anatomy of melancholia. Annu Rev Med 49:341–361, 1998

Drevets WC, Price JL, Simpson JR Jr, et al: Subgenual prefrontal cortex abnormalities in mood disorders. Nature 386:824–827, 1997

Elliott R, Sahakian BJ, McKay AP, et al: Neuropsychological impairments in unipolar depression: the influence of perceived failure on subsequent performance. Psychol Med 26(5):975–989, 1996

Elliott R, Friston KJ, Dolan RJ: Dissociable neural responses in human reward systems. J Neurosci 20:6159–6165, 2000

Ewart CK, Kolodner KB: Negative affect, gender, and expressive style predict elevated ambulatory blood pressure in adolescents. J Pers Soc Psychol 66:596–605, 1994

Feehan M, McGee R, Williams SM, et al: Mental health disorders from age 15 to age 18 years. J Am Acad Child Adolesc Psychiatry 32:1118–1126, 1993

Frith C: In what context is latent inhibition relevant to the symptoms of schizophrenia? Behav Brain Sci 14:28–29, 1991

Gauthier I, Tarr MJ, Anderson A, et al: Activation of the middle fusiform "face area" increases expertise in recognizing novel objects. Nat Neurosci 2:568–573, 1999

Giedd JN, Blumenthal J, Jeffries NO, et al: Brain development during adolescence: a longitudinal MRI study. Nat Neurosci 10:861–863, 1999

Goldstein RB, Weissman MM, Adams PB, et al: Psychiatric disorders in relatives of probands with panic disorder and/or major depression. Arch Gen Psychiatry 51:383–394, 1994

Hariri AR, Bookheimer SY, Mazziotta JC: Modulating emotional responses: effects of a neocortical network on the limbic system. Neuroreport 11:43–48, 2000

Henson R, Shallice T, Dolan R: Neuroimaging evidence for dissociable forms of repetition priming. Science. 287(5456):1269–1272, 2000

Irwin W, Davidson RJ, Lowe MJ, et al: Human amygdala activation detected with echo-planar functional magnetic resonance imaging. Neuroreport 7:1765–1769, 1996

Isenberg N, Silbersweig D, Engelien A, et al: Linguistic threat activates the human amygdala. Proc Natl Acad Sci U S A 96:10456–10459, 1999

Ishai A, Ungerleider LG, Martin A, et al: Distributed representation of objects in the human ventral visual pathway. Proc Nat Acad Sci U S A 96:9379–9384, 1999

Kagan, J: Galen's Prophecy. New York, Basic Books, 1995

Kanwisher N, McDermott J, Chun MM: The fusiform face area: a module in human extrastriate cortex specialized for face perception. J Neurosci 17:4302–4311, 1997

Karmiloff-Smith A: Development itself is the key to understanding developmental disorders. Trends in Cognitive Sciences 2:389–398, 1998

Keating DP: Adolescent thinking, in At the Threshold: The Developing Adolescent. Edited by Feldman SS, Elliott GR. Cambridge, MA, Harvard University Press, 1990, pp 54–92

Keating DP, Sasse DK: Cognitive socialization in adolescence: critical period for a critical habit of mind, in Psychosocial Development During Adolescence: Progress in Developmental contextualism. Edited by Adams GR, Montemayor R, Gullota TP. Thousand Oaks, CA, Sage, 1996, pp 232–258

Kentgen LM, Tencke CE, Pine DS, et al: A qEEG study of adolescent mood and anxiety disorders J Abnorm Psychol (in press)

Klein RG, Pine DS: Anxiety disorders, in Child and Adolescent Psychiatry: Modern Approaches, 3rd Edition. Edited by Rutter M, Taylor E. London, Blackwell Scientific Publications (in press)

Kolb B: Synaptic plasticity and the organization of behavior after early and late brain injury. Can J Exp Psychol 53:62–75, 1999

LaBar KS, Gatenby JC, Gore JC, et al: Human amygdala activation during conditioned fear acquisition and extinction: a mixed-trial fMRI study. Neuron 20:937–945, 1998

Lang PL, Bradley MM, Cuthbert BN: Emotion, motivation and anxiety: brain mechanisms and psychophysiology. Biol Psychiatry 44:1248–1263, 1998

LeDoux JE: The Emotional Brain. New York, Simon and Schuster, 1996

LeDoux JE: Fear and the brain: where have we been; where we are going? Biol Psychiatry 44:1229–1238, 1998

Lundh LG, Ost LG: Recognition for critical faces in social phobics. Behav Res Ther 34:787–794, 1996

MacDonald AW, Cohen JD, Stenger VA, et al: Dissociating the role of the dorsolateral prefrontal and anterior cingulate cortex in cognitive control. Science 288:1835–1838, 2000

Mathews A, MacLoed C: Cognitive approaches to emotion and emotional disorders. Annu Rev Psychol 45:25–50, 1994

McClure EB: A meta-analytic review of sex differences in facial expression processing and their development in infants, children, and adolescents. Psych Bull 126:424–453, 2000

McGlashan TH, Hoffman RE: Schizophrenia as a disorder of developmentally reduced synaptic connectivity. Arch Gen Psychiatry 57: 637–648, 2000

McNally RJ: Cognitive bias in the anxiety disorders. Nebr Symp Motiv 43:211–50, 1996

McNally RJ: Memory and anxiety disorders. Philos Trans R Soc London B Biol Sci 352:1755–1759, 1997

Merikangas KR, Avenevoli S, Dierker L, et al: Vulnerability factors among children at risk for anxiety disorders. Biol Psychiatry 46:1523–1535, 1999

Mesulam MM: From sensation to cognition. Brain 121:1013–1052, 1998

Mineka S, Sutton SK: Cognitive biases and the emotional disorders. Psychol Science 3:65–69, 1992

Mogg K, Bradley BP: A cognitive-motivational analysis of anxiety. Behav Res Ther 36:809–848, 1998

Mogg K, Bradley BP: Some methodological issues in assessing attentional biases for threatening faces in anxiety: a replication study using a modified version of the probe detection task. Behav Res Ther 37:595–604, 1999

Mori E, Ikeda M, Hirono N, et al: Amygdala volume and emotional memory in Alzheimer's disease. Am J Psychiatry 156:216–222, 1999

Murphy FC, Sahakian BJ, Rubinsztein JS, et al: Emotional bias and inhibitory control processes in mania and depression. Psychol Med 29:1307–1321, 1999

Nelson CA, Monk CS, Lin J, et al: Functional neuroanatomy of spatial working memory in children. Dev Psychol 36:109–116, 2000

Paus T, Zijdenbos A, Worsley K, et al: Structural maturation of neural pathways in children and adolescents: in vivo study. Science 283: 1908–1911, 1999

Peterson BS, Skudlarski P, Gatenby JC, et al: An fMRI study of Stroop word-color interference: evidence for cingulate subregions subserving multiple distributed attentional systems. Biol Psychiatry 45: 1237–1258, 1999

Phelps EA, Anderson AK: Emotional memory: what does the amygdala do? Curr Biol 7:R311–R314, 1997

Phillips ML, Young A, Senior C, et al: A specific neural substrate for perceiving disgust. Nature 389:495–498, 1997

Phillips ML, Bullmore ET, Howard R, et al: Investigation of facial recognition memory and happy and sad facial expression perception: an fMRI study. Psychiatry Res Sep 83(3):127–138, 1998

Pine DS, Cohen P, Gurley D, et al: The risk for early adulthood anxiety and depressive disorders in adolescents with anxiety and depressive disorders. Arch Gen Psychiatry 55:56–64, 1998

Pine DS, Cohen E, Cohen P, et al: Adolescent depressive symptoms as predictors of adult depression: moodiness or mood disorder? Am J Psychiatry 156:133–135, 1999a

Pine DS, Wasserman G, Wolk S: Memory and anxiety in pre-pubertal boys at risk for delinquency. J Am Acad Child Adolesc Psychiatry 38:1024–1031, 1999b

Pine DS, Kentgen LM, Bruder GE, et al: Cerebral laterality and adolescent depression. Psychiatry Res 93:135–144, 2000

Pine DS, Grun J, Peterson BS: Mapping brain circuits in developmental psychopathology: ADHD and anxiety as examples, in Brain Imaging. Edited by Rausch S, Dorrity D. Washington, DC, American Psychiatric Publishing (in press)

Ploghous A, Tracey I, Gati JS, et al: Dissociating pain from its anticipation in the human brain. Science 284:1979–1981, 1999

Robins, LN: Sturdy childhood predictors of adult antisocial behaviour: replications from longitudinal studies. Psychol Med 8:611–622, 1978

Rogers RD, Owen AM, Middleton HC, et al: Choosing between small, likely rewards and large, unlikely rewards activates inferior and orbital prefrontal cortex. J Neurosci 19:9029–9038, 1999

Rolls ET: The Brain and Emotion. New York, Oxford University Press, 1999

Rosenberg DR, Keshavan MS, O'Hearn KM, et al: Fronto-striatal measurement of treatment naïve pediatric obsessive compulsive disorders. Arch Gen Psychiatry 54:824–830, 1997

Schneider F, Weiss U, Kessler C, et al: Subcortical correlates of differential classical conditioning of aversive emotional reactions in social phobia. Biol Psychiatry 45:863–871, 1999

Schwartz CE, Snidman N, Kagan J: Adolescent social anxiety as an outcome of inhibited temperament in childhood. J Am Acad Child Adolesc Psychiatry 38:1008–1015, 1999

Sheline YI, Wang PW, Gado MH, et al: Hippocampal atrophy in recurrent major depression. Proc Natl Acad Sci U S A 30:3908–3913, 1996

Snowdon DA, Kemper SJ, Mortimer JA, et al: Linguistic ability in early life and cognitive function and Alzheimer's disease in late life: findings from the Nun Study. JAMA 275:528–532, 1996

Sowell ER, Thompson PM, Homes CJ, et al: In vivo evidence for post-adolescent brain maturation in frontal and striatal regions. Nat Neurosci 2:859–861, 1999

Squire LR, Kandel ER: Memory: From Mind to Molecules. New York, Scientific American Library, 1999

Staal WG, Hulshoff HE, Schnack HG, et al: Structural brain abnormalities in patients with schizophrenia and their healthy siblings. Am J Psychiatry 157:416–421, 2000

Steingard RJ, Renshaw PF, Yurgelun-Todd D, et al: Structural abnormalities in brain magnetic resonance images of depressed children. J Am Acad Child Adolesc Psychiatry 35:307–311, 1996

Szeszko PR, Robinson D, Alvir JM, et al: Orbital frontal and amygdala volume reductions in obsessive-compulsive disorder. Arch Gen Psychiatry 56:913–919, 1999

Taghavi MR, Neshat-Doost HT, Moradi AR, et al: Biases in visual attention in children and adolescents with clinical anxiety and mixed depression. J Abnorm Child Psychol 27:215–223, 1999

Teasdale JD, Howard RJ, Cox SG, et al: Functional MRI study of the cognitive generation of affect. Am J Psychiatry 156:209–215, 1999

Thomas KM, King SW, Franzen PL, et al: A developmental functional MRI study of spatial working memory. NeuroImage 10:327–338, 1999

Thomas KM, Eccard CH, Drevets WC, et al: Amygdala response to facial expressions in children and adults. J Cogn Neurosci (suppl):82B, 2000

Thompson PM, Giedd JN, Woods RP, et al: Growth patterns in the developing brain detected by using continuum mechanical tensor maps. Nature 404:190–193, 2000

Vasey MW, El-Hag N, Daleiden EL: Anxiety and the processing of emotionally stimuli: patterns of selective attention among high- and low-test anxious children. Child Dev 67:1173–1185, 1996

Weissman MM, Warner V, Wickramaratne P, et al: Offspring of depressed parents: 10 years later. Arch Gen Psychiatry 54:932–940, 1997

Whalen PJ. Fear, vigilance, and ambiguity: initial neuroimaging studies of the human amygdala. Current Directions in Psychological Science 7:177–187, 1998

Whalen PJ, Rauch SL, Etcoff JL, et al: Masked presentation of emotional facial expressions modulate amygdala activity without explicit knowledge. J Neurosci 18:411–418, 1998

Williams JMG, Mathews A, MacLoed C: The emotional Stroop task and psychopathology. Psycho Bull 120:3–24, 1996

Wright IC, Rabe-Hesketh S, Woodruff PWR, et al: Meta-analysis of regional brain volumes in schizophrenia. Am J Psychiatry 157:16–25, 2000

Zakzanis KK, Leach L, Kaplan E: On the nature and pattern of neu-rocognitive function in major depressive disorder. Neuropsychiatry Neuropsychol Behav Neurol 11:111–119, 1998

Zalla T, Koechlin E, Pietrini P, et al: Differential amygdala responses to winning and losing: a functional magnetic resonance imaging study in humans. Eur J Neurosci 12:1764–1770, 2000

Chapter 4

Brain Structure and Function in Late-Life Depression

Harold A. Sackeim, Ph.D.

The risk for depressive syndromes is lifelong. The diagnosis and treatment of depressive disorders in the elderly can be particularly difficult, given underreporting or minimization of symptoms, comorbid medical conditions, and other factors (Lebowitz et al. 1997). Depression in late life is often viewed as a natural consequence of the aging process and attributed to psychological reactions to medical infirmity and the loss of social support and job roles. However, there is compelling evidence that late-life depression is characterized by abnormalities of brain structure and functional brain activity that cannot be explained by the normal aging process. Indeed, there is evidence in some domains that individuals who have their first major depression late in life (late-onset illness) have more profound structural and functional brain disturbances than patients with early-onset illness. This suggests that biological dysregulation may be responsible for many of the depressive syndromes manifested with aging. In turn, our understanding of the nature of these biological abnormalities is leading to new perspectives on the prevention, diagnosis, and treatment of late-life depression.

Preparation of this chapter was supported in part by grant MH55646 from the National Institute of Mental Health, Bethesda, MD.

Brain Structural Abnormalities: Encephalomalacia

In comparison to healthy control subjects and other neuropsychiatric groups, high rates of abnormality have been consistently observed in magnetic resonance imaging (MRI) evaluations of elderly patients with major depressive disorder (MDD; see Sackeim et al. 2000 for a review). These abnormalities appear as areas of increased signal intensity in balanced (mixed T_1- and T_2-weighted), T_2-weighted, and fluid-attenuated inversion recovery (FLAIR) images. T_1-weighted sequences maximize the contrast between gray and white matter and provide fine anatomic detail. In contrast, T_2-weighted and FLAIR sequences are particularly sensitive in identifying fluid-filled areas, which appear as areas of high signal intensity. Abnormalities can be classified into three types: 1) *Periventricular hyperintensities* (PVHs) are halos or rims adjacent to ventricles; in severe forms, these invade surrounding deep white matter. 2) Alternatively, single, patchy, or confluent foci may be observed in subcortical white matter, with or without PVH; these are *deep white matter hyperintensities* (DWMHs). 3) *Hyperintensities* (HIs) may also be found in deep gray structures, particularly the basal ganglia, thalamus, and pons. Collectively, these three types of abnormality have been referred to as *leukoencephalopathy, leukoaraiosis, subcortical arteriosclerotic encephalopathy, encephalomalacia,* and *unidentified bright objects.* Since HI in MDD is not restricted to white matter and its etiology is not established, the term *encephalomalacia* is used here to refer to all three types of abnormality.

Figure 4–1 illustrates a moderate-to-severe case of encephalomalacia. FLAIR images are presented from a patient with late-onset, first-episode major depression treated at the Late-Life Depression Clinic of the New York State Psychiatric Institute. The image on the left illustrates PVH, with thick bands of high signal intensity (white) adjacent to the lateral ventricles. Note that, on the left side of this image, the HIs extend into the deep white matter. The image on the right is a higher MRI slice from the same patient, and shows multiple confluent HIs in the deep white matter (i.e., DWMHs). As discussed below, in patients presenting with

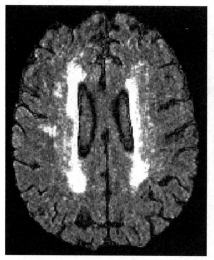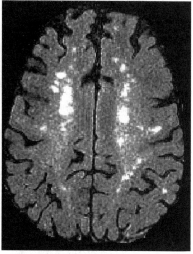

Figure 4–1. Magnetic resonance imaging (MRI) fluid-attenuated inversion recovery images of a patient with late-onset major depression. Bright areas show MRI hyperintensities. The image on the left demonstrates periventricular hyperintensities, with a broad band of increased signal adjacent to the lateral ventricles and invading the deep white matter. The image on the right, from the same patient at a higher level, shows multiple, confluent foci of hyperintensities in the deep white matter (centrum semiovale).

these MRI findings clinicians typically receive radiological reports that emphasize small vessel disease.

In one of the largest prospective MRI studies of late-life major depression, all 51 elderly patients (age > 60 years) referred for electroconvulsive therapy (ECT) presented with HI, with over half rated as moderate to severe, and 51% had lesions of subcortical gray nuclei (Coffey et al. 1990). These rates of abnormality greatly exceeded those found in a healthy control sample, with basal ganglia abnormalities most discriminative (see Figure 4–2). The depressed samples studied to date have often included patients with comorbid medical illnesses, without adequate control for cerebrovascular disease (CVD) risk factors, medications, or drug abuse. Nonetheless, in the report by Coffey et al. (1990), even when MDD patients with preexisting neurological conditions were excluded the rate of encephalomalacia greatly exceeded

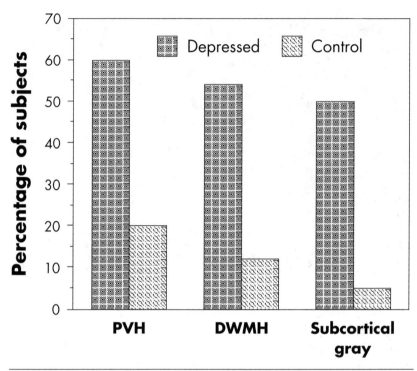

Figure 4–2.   A representation of the findings of Coffey et al. (1990). Percentage rates of periventricular hyperintensity (PVH), deep white matter hyperintensity (DWMH), and hyperintensities in subcortical gray matter structures are contrasted for patients with major depression and control subjects.

that of normal control subjects. In a replication study, MDD patients had marked increases in the frequency of PVH, DWMH, and basal ganglia and thalamic HI relative to control subjects matched for CVD risk factors (Coffey et al. 1993). The age-adjusted odds ratio for PVH was 5.32. In other (often large) population studies of elderly healthy control subjects, when the halos or caps commonly found at the top and bottom of the lateral ventricles are excluded it is found that approximately 10%–30% of psychiatrically healthy subjects present with MRI white-matter abnormalities (with typically mild severity) and with low rates of subcortical gray matter abnormalities (e.g., Breteler et al. 1994b).

The rate or severity of encephalomalacia in geriatric depression may equal or exceed that in Alzheimer's disease (Erkinjuntti et al. 1994) and may be comparable to that in multi-infarct dementia (e.g., Zubenko et al. 1990; see Sackeim et al. 2000 for a review). In considerably younger samples, several groups have reported that HIs are more common among young bipolar patients than among control subjects (Dupont et al. 1990, 1995; Swayze et al. 1990). Aylward et al. (1994) found that older (>38 years), not younger, bipolar patients had an excess of HI. Brown et al. (1992) did not detect an excess in young bipolar patients, although they did observe that severe HI was overrepresented in elderly patients with MDD.

Clinical Correlates

We are beginning to understand the clinical and historical features of depressive illness associated with encephalomalacia. Coffey et al. (1990, 1993) suggested that medication-resistant patients with late-onset MDD (onset ≥60 years) are at increased risk. The patients in these studies were consecutive referrals to an ECT service and were unusual in that the rate of late-onset depression was 80%, with 86% said to be medication resistant. However, in this study the criteria for medication resistance were not consistent with modern standards for medication dosage and duration and included medication-intolerant patients.

Age at Onset

A number of studies have found an association between encephalomalacia and age at onset of illness. Lesser et al. (1991) reported an excess of large DWMH in patients with late-onset psychotic depression compared with psychiatrically and neurologically healthy subjects. Figiel et al. (1991) found that a higher rate of caudate HI and large DWMH distinguished late-onset from early-onset MDD in a small sample of unipolar patients. In a larger sample, Hickie et al. (1995) found that late age at onset and negative family history of mood disorder were associated with more severe DWMH. In relatively small samples of elderly MDD patients and control subjects with equivalent frequency of CVD risk factors, Krishnan et al. (1993) found that late-onset illness was associated with smaller volumes of the caudate and lenticular nuclei and greater frequency and severity of DWMH. In a subsequent study, Krishnan et al. (1997) compared 32 elderly MDD patients with encephalomalacia to 57 MDD patients without encephalomalacia. Controlling for age, the group characterized by MRI abnormalities had later age at onset and tended to have a lower rate of positive family history for mood disorder. Lesser et al. (1996) also found that, independent of current age, patients with late-onset MDD had larger areas of white-matter HI than patients with early-onset (<35 years) recurrent MDD. Fujiwaka et al. (1994) found a higher rate of "silent cerebral infarctions" in late-onset compared to early-onset MDD. Patients with these large HIs also had a lower rate of family history of mood disorder. Dahabra et al. (1998) compared small groups of early- and late-onset elderly patients who had recovered from an episode of MDD. White matter HIs were more common in the late-onset group, as was ventricular enlargement. Salloway et al. (1996) compared 15 MDD late-onset (≥60 years) MDD patients to 15 early-onset (<60 years) MDD patients using semiautomated measures of DWMH and PVH area. A marked difference was observed, with the late-onset group having twice the subcortical HI of the early-onset group. O'Brien et al. (1996) also reported that DWMHs were most common in severely ill inpatients with late-onset MDD.

Thus, a large number of independent investigations have seen either higher prevalence or severity of encephalomalacia in late-onset depression than in early-onset depression, with few negative findings (Dupont et al. 1995; Ebmeier et al. 1997; Greenwald et al. 1996). There is also a suggestion, less consistently observed, that MDD patients with these MRI abnormalities are less likely to have a positive family history for mood disorder.

Severity and Nature of Depressive Symptoms

With the exceptions of Lesser et al. (1994) and Kumar et al. (1998), MRI research has generally focused on inpatients with severe symptoms, often referred for ECT. Generalizability to the far more common phenomenon of MDD in outpatients needs to be established, particularly since symptom severity has not been found to correlate with encephalomalacia. There is also no indication of a difference in rate or severity of encephalomalacia between psychotic and nonpsychotic depression. In fact, Krishnan et al. (1997) reported that patients with encephalomalacia were less likely to have psychotic symptoms, though more likely to present with anhedonia. Phenomenological differences as a function of encephalomalacia have rarely been examined.

Treatment Response and Long-Term Outcome

Coffey et al. (1990) suggested that patients with encephalomalacia show positive response to ECT, but improvement was evaluated retrospectively and globally. In contrast, Hickie et al. (1995) reported that severity of DWMH predicted poorer outcome with either heterogeneous pharmacological regimens or ECT. In a retrospective study, Fujikawa et al. (1996) found that patients with severe silent cerebral infarction (both perforating and in cortical areas) had longer hospital stays and poorer response to antidepressant medications than MDD patients without infarction. In a study of 44 MDD patients between 65 and 85 years of age, Simpson et al. (1997) found that globally assessed short-term clinical outcome was poorer in patients with DWMH and HI in the basal ganglia or pons. To date, there has been no prospective evaluation of the prognostic significance of these structural abnormalities using a standardized pharmacological protocol. The available evidence is consistent, however, in suggesting that encephalomalacia is associated with poorer short-term response to antidepressant treatments. Given these findings, particularly aggressive treatment regimens may be needed in patients with significant encephalomalacia.

In a sample of 37 patients followed for an average of 14 months, Hickie et al. (1997) provided the first evidence that DWMH in MDD predicts poor long-term outcome. DWMH, late age at onset, and cerebrovascular risk factors were linked to chronic depression and cognitive decline, with a subgroup developing vascular dementia. The linkage between poor outcome and encephalomalacia was supported in another recent study. O'Brien et al. (1998) followed 60 MDD patients over 55 years of age for an average of 32 months. Time to relapse with depressive symptoms or cognitive decline was the outcome measure. Patients with severe white matter HI at baseline had a median survival time of only 136 days, in contrast to 315 days for those without severe HI. In light of the recurrent and often chronic nature of MDD and given the evidence that depressive symptoms in the elderly may be prodromal to dementing conditions, further investigation of the prognostic significance of encephalomalacia is clearly needed.

Adverse Side Effects

Elderly MDD patients with basal ganglia HI may be prone to develop delirium when treated with antidepressant medications or ECT (Figiel et al. 1989, 1990). However, this work, based on small samples, did not examine the specificity of the relation to encephalomalacia in other subcortical or white-matter areas. Fujikawa et al. (1996) retrospectively assessed the relationship of silent cerebral infarction to adverse effects and response to pharmacotherapy in MDD patients over the age of 50. Patients with silent infarctions had a higher incidence of central nervous system adverse events, and the frequency of adverse events increased with the severity of infarction.

Cognition and Neurological Signs

In psychiatrically and neurologically healthy, nonsymptomatic subjects some degree of encephalomalacia may be observed, and its prevalence and extent is linked to aging. It is unclear whether the limited encephalomalacia in medically healthy samples is associated with cognitive impairment, and there may be threshold effects for HI volume (Boone et al. 1992). Nonetheless, in medically healthy and neurological samples there is a concentration of replicated findings specifically associating encephalomalacia with deficits in attention, motor speed, and executive function (e.g., Breteler et al. 1994a; see Sackeim et al. 2000 for a review). These are hallmark areas of deficit in MDD in the elderly (Sackeim and Steif, 1988). In nonpsychiatric patient samples, the most common neurological abnormalities associated with encephalomalacia are gait disturbances, tendency to fall, extensor plantar reflex, and other primitive reflexes.

Surprisingly, there has been limited investigation of the neuropsychological correlates of encephalomalacia in MDD. Ebmeier et al. (1997) found that severity of DWMH was inversely related to global cognitive function (as measured by Mini-Mental State Exam scores) in elderly patients with MDD. In the most comprehensive study to date, Lesser et al. (1996) contrasted 60 late-onset (≥50 years) MDD patients, 35 early-onset (<35 years) MDD patients, and 165 psychiatrically healthy control subjects. All subjects were at least 50 years of age. The late-onset group had greater DWMH than either of the other groups. Cognitive deficits were most marked in the late-onset group and pertained to nonverbal intelligence, nonverbal memory, constructional ability, executive function, and speed of processing. Patients with greater severity of DWMH had significantly poorer executive function.

Jenkins et al. (1998) found that elderly MDD patients with HI showed poorer performance on a number of learning and memory indices, with the pattern of deficits resembling that in subcortical degenerative disorders (i.e., Huntington's and Parkinson's diseases). Simpson et al. (1997) conducted neuropsychological assessment following treatment of an elderly MDD sample. Hyperintensities in the pons were associated with reduced psychomotor speed, basal ganglia HIs were linked to impaired category productivity (executive function), and PVHs were associated with recall deficits. Since the severity of encephalomalacia in this study was also associated with clinical outcome, the findings regarding neuropsychological correlates may have been confounded with clinical state. There is a need for comprehensive neuropsychological and neurological evaluations of elderly MDD patients in relation to structural and functional imaging deficits.

Etiology of Encephalomalacia

Neuropathology: Linkage to Cerebrovascular Disease

The pathogenesis of the MRI abnormalities in MDD is unknown. In non-MDD samples these abnormalities usually have been attributed to ischemic CVD, with HI reflecting increased water content in perivascular space, axon and myelin loss, astrocyte proliferation (gliosis), and/or frank infarction (Awad et al. 1986a; Chimowitz et al. 1992; van Swieten et al. 1991; see Sackeim et al. 2000 for a review). Typically, the HIs are in watershed areas supplied by small arterioles that branch off long, penetrating medullary and lenticulostriate arteries. These areas receive limited collateral supply and are particularly vulnerable to vascular insult. In all the populations studied, including MDD and medically healthy control subjects, age has been the most critical correlate. To a lesser extent, these abnormalities are also associated with hypertension, diabetes, coronary heart disease, and other vascular risk factors (e.g., Awad et al. 1986c; Breteler et al. 1994b; Coffey et al. 1990).

In a study of patients with Alzheimer's disease, frank CVD at one year follow-up was observed only in those patients with baseline computerized tomography (CT) white matter lucencies (Lopez et al. 1992). In 215 patients with lacunar infarction, prospective 3-year follow-up indicated that baseline encephalomalacia predicted subsequent stroke, new-onset dementia, and death (Miyao et al. 1992). Several other studies have indicated that encephalomalacia predicts subsequent stroke, myocardial infarction, and vascular death (e.g., Tarvonen-Schroder et al. 1995). Boiten et al. (1993) found a considerably higher rate of encephalomalacia in patients with asymptomatic lacunar infarcts than in patients with symptomatic lacunar infarcts (odds ratio: 10.7). These groups differed in the location and implicated vascular territories of the infarcts, with the suggestion offered that ischemia due to arteriosclerosis leads to encephalomalacia and silent lacunar infarcts, while microatheromatosis more commonly produces symptomatic lacunar infarcts. There is also evidence of greater 24-hour variability in blood pressure among patients with HI, suggesting periodic ischemic compromise.

Induction of similar T_2-weighted abnormalities in animals is now done via middle cerebral artery occlusion. Awad et al. (1993) reported the first prospective de novo appearance of DWMH in humans. Despite full anticoagulation, four of eight patients undergoing therapeutic inferior carotid artery occlusion (detachable balloon technique) developed ipsilateral subcortical HI. Thus, a large array of findings supports a vascular etiology.

Awad et al.'s (1986c) suggestion of état criblé is also compatible with the data. Pulsation in ectatic or tortuous blood vessels rigidified by sclerosis may mechanically increase water-filled perivascular space, with parenchymal atrophy resulting from ischemic substrate supply. Some types of PVH may be due to cerebrospinal fluid (CSF) leakage into surrounding tissue. Caps at the horns of the lateral ventricles are common in psychiatrically healthy individuals, may not be age-related, and may be due to interstitial flow into ventricles, combined with low myelin content and ependymitis granularis. Therefore, including caps in encephalomalacia ratings can lead to high false-positive rates.

There has been considerable histopathological investigation of HI, but not in MDD. The findings generally support a vascular etiology, as areas of HI in patients with neurological disease and medically healthy samples commonly show arteriolar hyalinization, ectasia, enlarged perivascular (Virchow-Robin) space, gliosis, spongiosis, and/or lacunar infarcts (Awad et al. 1986c; Chimowitz et al. 1992). Van Swieten et al. (1991) found that DWMHs were invariably accompanied by demyelination and gliosis and less consistently with increased perivascular space. The demyelination was strongly associated with increased wall thickness of small arterioles. They concluded that arteriosclerosis in small arterioles (<150 μm) is the primary cause, leading to demyelination and then cell loss with progression. Munoz et al. (1993) suggested that some pathological changes could also be due to microaneurysms at the points of arteriole bifurcation, resulting in leakage of serum proteins (edema). Fazekas et al. (1993) observed that the size and appearance of MRI-defined PVH and DWMH were strongly associated with the extent of ischemic tissue damage. Moody et al. (1995) offered the novel finding that venous collagenosis is strongly associated with encephalomalacia. They found marked thickening of periventricular postcapillary venules and collecting veins that provide drainage of the centrum semiovale and suggested that disordered venous drainage results in distal chronic ischemia and brain edema

The notion that late-life depression is associated with ischemic vascular disease was recently supported in a postmortem study of the expression of intercellular adhesion molecule-1 (ICAM-1).

ICAM-1 is a vascular marker of inflammation, whose expression is increased by ischemia. Thomas et al. (2000) assayed ICAM-1 in the dorsolateral prefrontal cortex (DLPFC) and occipital cortex in 20 deceased individuals over the age of 60 with a history of MDD and in 20 comparison subjects with no history of MDD. Expression of ICAM-1 was significantly greater in DLPFC gray and white matter of the depressed group with no difference in occipital cortex. This finding, in addition to reinforcing the vascular hypothesis for late-life depression, is compatible with the well-replicated finding that the DLPFC is a common site for reduced regional cerebral blood flow (rCBF) and regional cerebral metabolic rate for glucose ($rCMR_{glu}$) in MDD (see below).

Pathophysiology of Encephalomalacia

One way of testing the view that encephalomalacia reflects local ischemic damage is to quantify rCBF and other metabolic processes in areas of HI. No study has co-registered functional and structural images and quantified perfusion or metabolism in the areas of asymptomatic MRI-defined HI. Such research is in progress by our group. However, in recent years, at least 20 studies have examined more general perfusion or metabolic abnormalities in samples characterized by extent of encephalomalacia.

Meguro et al. (1990) conducted one of the key studies, using positron emission tomography (PET) with the ^{15}O-PET steady-state method to quantify rCBF, regional cerebral metabolic rate for oxygen ($rCMRO_2$), regional oxygen extraction fraction (rOEF), and regional cerebral blood volume (rCBV) in 28 asymptomatic individuals with CVD risk factors. More severe PVH was associated with global reductions in gray-matter CBF and in the CBF/CBV ratio, with the latter parameter free of partial volume effects. In contrast, OEF tended to increase with severe PVH, and global CMRO2 only tended to be reduced with increasing PVH. These effects were consistent across gray-matter regions and suggested a compensatory mismatch between metabolism and CBF ("misery perfusion"). That is, as CBF (tissue perfusion) declined, OEF (oxygen extraction) increased to maintain metabolic rate. De Reuck et al. (1992), also using the ^{15}O-PET steady-state method, reported similar findings. White-matter CT lucencies were associated with lowered CBF in frontal and parietal gray and white matter, in both demented and normal subjects. Particularly in frontal white matter, encephalomalacia was associated with increased OEF, with greater reductions in rCBF than in $rCMRO_2$. Similarly, Hatazawa et al. (1997) compared 8 normal subjects without encephalomalacia and 15 asymptomatic individuals with white-matter HI using $H_2^{15}O$-, $C^{15}O$-, and $^{15}O_2$-PET. White-matter HIs were associated with reduced CBF and increased OEF in the cerebral white matter and basal ganglia, without effects in the thalamus.

In the only similar study in MDD, Lesser et al. (1994) reported that patients with large areas of white-matter HI tended to have the greatest deficits in whole-brain CBF. Of note, in this elderly sample (>60 years) whole-brain CBF was markedly diminished across the MDD group and the subgroup with HI had the largest deficit.

Promoting vasodilatation through the use of a hypercapnic challenge may be a particularly useful method for investigating the pathophysiology of encephalomalacia. Brown et al. (1990), using stable xenon CT, found that, compared to control subjects, CVD patients with encephalomalacia had diminished white-matter CBF response to acetazolamide. In 28 asymptomatic subjects, Isaka et al. (1997) found that the extent of PVH was marginally related to global gray-matter resting CBF ($r = -0.36$) but strongly related to global CBF after hypercapnic challenge with acetazolamide ($r = -0.78$), as well as to the CBF change between rest and hypercapnia ($r = -0.57$). This study linked PVH in asymptomatic individuals to a diffuse reduction in cerebrovascular dilatory capacity (i.e., hemodynamic reserve), suggesting that small-vessel disease may not only characterize the territories of the subcortical HI but may be widespread in the cortical gray matter as well. Similarly, in a study using ^{99}Tc hexamethyl propyleneamine oxime (HMPAO) single photon emission computer tomography (SPECT) in patients with unilateral carotid occlusive disease, severity of DWMH and PVH were linked to perfusion deficits at rest, with the associations magnified following acetazolamide (hypercapnic) challenge (Isaka et al. 1997).

Virtually all 20 of the studies that have examined perfusion or metabolic abnormalities in samples (only one with MDD) characterized by extent of encephalomalacia found relations between white-matter HI and measures of perfusion. While CBF deficits in white matter were common, diffuse cortical gray-matter deficits were also observed. Findings have consistently linked encephalomalacia to low CBF and increased OEF, suggesting that the relations between the structural and functional deficits are more marked for perfusion than metabolism measures. This has been observed in work assessing both CBF and $CMRO_2$ or CMR_{glu}. It is not known if such uncoupling occurs in geriatric depression. Indeed, it is almost invariably assumed that rCBF deficits in mood disorders reflect disturbed patterns of neuronal activity and not a constrained vascular substrate. In contrast, the hypothesis can now be raised that this assumption is false in late life, or specifically in late-onset depression, and that deficits are greater for global CBF than for global CMR. Further, findings linking encephalomalacia to reduced CBF response to hypercapnia suggest both that limited vasodilatory capacity may be an important correlate and that structure/function relations become magnified with hypercapnic (vasodilatory) challenge.

Longitudinal Perspective

Across populations, cross-sectional studies have all indicated that the likelihood and severity of encephalomalacia increase with age. In addition, the possibility that encephalomalacia and perfusion deficits in MDD are progressive is suggested by the associations with CVD risk factors, the follow-up results in neurologic disease samples indicate increased rates of future CVD, functional compromise, and death as a function of baseline encephalomalacia, the histopathological findings in the areas containing HI, and the hypothesis of underlying ischemic CVD. Clearly, it is important to determine whether the MRI abnormalities are progressive, reflecting a degenerative disease pattern. Several groups are now conducting MRI studies examining change in encephalomalacia at long-term follow-up in late-life patients with MDD. However, the only data reported to date are limited to an examination of MDD patients before and 6 months following ECT (Coffey et al. 1991). Blind ratings showed strong test-retest stability in HI evaluations, with the only changes being a worsening of encephalomalacia in four patients. The follow-up interval was probably too short for MRI changes to be observed. In this context, perfusion imaging may provide more sensitive measures of progressive effects than MRI. If ischemia in deep structures leads to encephalomalacia, it should exist prior to MRI evidence of structural deficit and its quantification should be more sensitive to progressive change.

The findings regarding encephalomalacia in MDD are largely consistent. They suggest that ischemic small vessel disease leads to destruction of white-matter tracts and, in some cases, of subcortical nuclei. Anatomically, frontal-striatal circuits are most commonly implicated (Coffey et al. 1990; Greenwald et al. 1998).

Establishing that a progressive CVD process contributes to late-onset MDD should have important implications for understanding the phenomenology, prevention, and treatment of MDD. There is controversial evidence that in some patients the course of affective illness becomes more virulent with aging, with shorter periods of euthymia between episodes, more abrupt onset of acute symptoms, and greater resistance to treatment. Late-onset MDD may be particularly treatment resistant. Treatment of MDD often involves use of agents with potential cardiac and cerebrovascular effects (e.g., tricyclic antidepressants). Conceivably, some of these effects, such as hypotension and reductions in CBF or metabolism, may aggravate a CVD process and perhaps limit efficacy or enhance side effects. Thus, there is the possibility that some treatments that are effective in suppressing the expression of the acute depressive episode may in the long run contribute to disease progression. Finally, tying functional and structural abnormalities to a CVD process may suggest alternative methods of treatment and new approaches to disease prevention.

Volumetric Brain Structural Abnormalities

The earliest studies of structural brain abnormalities in psychiatric disorders concentrated on the area or volume of CSF-filled spaces, most commonly on the size of the lateral ventricles and on cortical sulcal widening (e.g., Weinberger et al. 1979). Particularly in the context of late-life depression, enlarged ventricles and sulcal widening have usually been interpreted as reflecting a nonspecific atrophic process resulting in the loss of brain tissue, as opposed to a developmental dysplasia reflecting abnormal brain growth.

Ventricular Enlargement and Sulcal Prominence

Scores of studies across the age span have tested whether patients with mood disorders have ventricular enlargement and increased sulcal prominence. Meta-analysis indicates that both are indeed the case, and that the ventricular enlargement observed in mood-disorder patients is of nearly the same magnitude as in patients with schizophrenia (Elkis et al. 1995). Thus, even outside the context of major depression in late life there is substantial evidence for loss of brain tissue. However, few studies of ventricular enlargement or sulcal prominence have focused on late-life depression. There is some evidence that ventricular enlargement may be especially prominent in late-onset relative to early-onset geriatric depression (Dahabra et al. 1998). This would reinforce the notion of an active atrophic process.

The possibility must be kept in mind that the evidence for an atrophic brain process in mood disorders could result from a variety of artifacts, including the effects of medications on brain structure. There is substantial evidence that lithium, tricyclic antidepressants, and perhaps monoamine oxidase inhibitors can produce fluid changes and alter cerebral microcirculation. There is the concern that antidepressant or antimanic medications may result in increased extracellular water content, which in turn may result in enlarged fluid-filled spaces, although very recent evidence suggests that treatment with lithium may actually lead to an increase in cerebral gray-matter content (Moore et al. 2000). While there is fairly compelling evidence that neuroleptic exposure is unrelated to ventricular enlargement in schizophrenia, the possible confounding effects of prior medications may be more difficult to rule out in mood disorders. This is of greatest concern in early-onset late-life depression, where patients will have the longest histories of exposure to psychotropic agents. Medication-naive depressed patients may often be younger, less severely ill, and perhaps less likely to manifest the relevant brain-structural phenomena. However, a variety of investigators have examined the role of medication history by correlating the type and length of previous medication exposure with imaging results. Universally, the results have been negative (see Sackein and Prohovnik 1993 for a review). At the same time, it must be recognized that retrospective quantification of lifetime medication exposure may have limited reliability and validity.

Age and Age at Onset

Cross-sectional studies suggest that in medically healthy individuals there appears to be little change in ventricular brain ratio (VBR), the most common measure of lateral ventricular enlargement, between approximately 20 and 60 years of age, while afterward there is a progressive increase. This pattern raises both methodological and conceptual concerns. From a methodological viewpoint, the pattern indicates that in normal healthy subjects the association between age and VBR is nonlinear. However, virtually all of the studies that have used age as a covariate in comparisons of mood-disorder patients with control subjects or with other psychiatric groups have treated this relation in a linear manner. Not only may this have resulted in decreased sensitivity in the comparisons (and higher rates of Type II error), but some of the reported findings may be misleading. For example, Dolan et al. (1985) are the only investigators to date to explicitly examine interaction effects on VBR between diagnosis of unipolar or bipolar depression and age of patients. This interaction achieved a significance level of 0.18, possibly supporting the conclusion that patients with unipolar depression and patients with bipolar depression may manifest ventricular enlargement at different age ranges (late in those with unipolar depression, early in those with bipolar depression); a more sensitive data analysis strategy might have revealed a more robust effect. Similarly, the interaction between status as mood-disorder patient (unipolar or bipolar) and age achieved a significance level of 0.14. However, as the authors commented, inspection of the data indicated that it was only in the older age groups that quantitative VBR differences were evident.

There are other suggestions in this literature of the importance of aging effects. Jacoby and Levy (1980), in a sample of 41 mood-disorder patients and 50 medically healthy control subjects, all over the age of 60, failed to find a difference in average VBR. They noted, however, that nine of the patients (22%) had evidence of ventricular enlargement and that this subgroup was characterized by later onset of illness, older age, and higher mortality at 2-year follow-up than the remaining patients. In a prospective longitudinal study of the community sample of Jacoby and Levy (1980), Bird et al. (1986) found that ventricular enlargement at baseline was predictive of development of late-onset depression.

In this light, it is conceivable that a subgroup of patients with late-onset depression, typically unipolar, may be especially likely to manifest ventricular enlargement, while ventricular enlargement may also characterize younger bipolar patients. If this were the case, cross-sectional comparison of unipolar and bipolar patients and normal control subjects in the younger age range would reveal enlarged VBR as characteristic of bipolar but not of unipolar disorder (e.g., Andreasen et al. 1990). At the same time, among older patients there may be no difference between patients with bipolar depression and those with unipolar depression (e.g., Dolan et al. 1985). This type of specification could prove valuable in contributing to our understanding of the etiology of VBR enlargement in mood disorders. Manifestation of enlarged VBR in younger patients is compatible with the view that ventriculomegaly may reflect neurodevelopmental dysplasia, in which case it should be nonprogressive. Manifestation of enlarged VBR primarily in older, late-onset patients is compatible with an atrophic process, which may or may not be progressive.

Phenomenology

Other than the distinction between psychotic and nonpsychotic illness, few phenomenological features of depression have been found to correlate significantly with VBR or other structural measures in more than one investigation. There have been surprisingly few attempts to associate VBR with overall severity of depressive illness, as assessed by instruments such as the Hamilton Rating Scale for Depression (HRSD). In the main, such attempts have produced negative results. Schlegel et al. (1989) reported that in 44 medication-free (nonelderly) depressed patients, VBR and width of the third ventricle were associated with scores on the Brief Psychiatric Rating Scale, Bech-Rafaelsen Melancholia Scale, Global Assessment Scale, Rating for Emotional Blunting, and Scale for Assessment of Negative Symptoms. At the same time, the structural measures were not associated with HRSD scores or scores on the Hamilton Rating Scale for Anxiety. Item analyses suggested that ventricular size was most associated with retardation-related items. They suggested that scales such as the HRSD may be too multidimensional to reveal consistent effect, particularly since anxiety symptoms and somatic complaints may obscure relations. For the most part, patient subtyping into "endogenous" and "nonendogenous" or "melancholic" and "nonmelancholic" categories has not revealed structural differences. Several investigators have sought associations between VBR or other brain morphometric measures and family history of psychiatric illness. No positive findings have been reported (see Sackein and Prohovnik 1993 for a review).

The significance of delusional or other psychotic symptoms in relation to ventricular enlargement is controversial. Larger VBR in psychotic mood-disorder patients has been reported by a number of investigators, but not by all; see Sackeim and Prohovnik (1993) for a review. The reasons for this inconsistency are poorly understood, but it should be noted that in many cases sample sizes have been small. Whatever contribution is made by mood disorders to VBR and related measures, that contribution is difficult to separate from the naturally occurring variability, which is substantial in medically healthy samples. When one adds to this the possibility that effects on VBR may be dependent on age group, gender, and/or other diagnostic subtyping (unipolar vs. bipolar), it is clear that power to detect effects was severely compromised in much of this literature.

Cognitive Status

Characteristically, during the acute phase of illness the performance of patients with major depression or mania is reduced on cognitive tests heavily influenced by the adequacy of attention and concentration (e.g., immediate learning and memory; Sackeim and Steif 1988). Furthermore, a small subgroup of patients with major depression shows more profound cognitive disturbance, with impaired orientation and global performance deficits in the range of demented patients. This constellation in depression is usually referred to as *pseudodementia* and is seen almost exclusively in late-life depression. In depressed samples not specifically selected for cognitive impairment there are scattered findings of inverse associations between VBR and specific cognitive measures, as well as a variety of negative findings; see Sackeim and Prohovnik (1993) for a review. For instance, there has been a report that degree of residual cognitive impairment following recovery from depression in an elderly sample was positively associated with VBR obtained 2 years earlier during the acute depressive phase (Abas et al. 1990).

Perhaps a more powerful methodology is to contrast structural findings in depressed patients with and without prominent cognitive impairment. Pearlson et al. (1989) identified 15 depressed patients who were cognitively impaired at admission and 11 patients who were unimpaired, using a cutoff of 24 on the Mini-Mental State Exam for this designation. These 26 depressed patients, all older than 60 years, were compared in CT measures to 13 patients with probable Alzheimer's disease and 31 medically health control subjects, all comparably aged. Of the cognitively impaired depressed patients, 11 were reexamined at 2-year follow-up and only one of this group evidenced cognitive decline. On CT measures of VBR and brain density, the total depressed sample fell between the Alzheimer's disease patients and control subjects. Specific comparisons indicated that, relative to the normal control subjects, VBR was larger and brain density was less in the cognitively impaired depressed group and in the Alzheimer's disease group. The cognitively intact depressed group did not differ from healthy control subjects. Related findings indicated that VBR and brain density measures were associated with neuropsychological performance variables only in the cognitively impaired groups. This study suggested that ventricular enlargement and possibly other structural abnormalities may be particularly manifest in elderly depressed patients with concurrent, reversible, and moderate-to-marked cognitive impairment.

Course of Illness

Correlations have been sought in samples unselected for age between many descriptive features of affective illness course with VBR and other brain morphometric measures. With some important exceptions, however, the findings have been either negative or isolated and unreplicated. It does not appear that duration of affective illness, duration of current episode, number of previous affective episodes, or number of previous psychiatric hospitalizations are related to structural abnormalities; see Sackeim and Prohovnik (1993) for a review. Acute to short-term response to treatment has also shown no relation to VBR. However, Jacoby and Levy (1980) observed that treatment response after 3 months did not distinguish elderly patients with and without ventricular enlargement. Nonetheless, there was a higher mortality rate in patients with such enlargement at 2-year follow-up. Shima et al. (1984) reported that larger VBR was associated with poorer clinical outcome 9 months after admission in elderly depressed patients. As noted above, Bird et al. (1986) suggested that baseline VBR in a community sample was predictive of the development of late-onset depression. Therefore, ventricular enlargement may have a prognostic significance in the elderly not seen in younger populations. Increased VBR in geriatric depression may be associated with late onset of illness, greater cognitive impairment (at least during the acute phase), poorer likelihood of recovery, and a higher rate of mortality.

Brain Structural Morphometry

With the development of high-resolution MRI and computerized techniques to segment brain tissue into gray, white, and CSF regions, the focus has shifted in recent years from measurement of CSF-filled spaces (e.g., of ventricular enlargement) to assessment of the volume of specific cerebral structures. Across the age span there is suggestive evidence for abnormal brain volume (decreased or increased) in mood-disorder patients in frontal cortex, temporal cortex, amygdala, hippocampus, corpus striatum, an area in medial prefrontal cortex just below the genu of the corpus callosum, and other structures. Little of this work has yet focused on late-life depression, even though all the foregoing information suggests that deficits most likely would be manifested here. Consequently, only a few relevant findings are emphasized below.

In a sample of relatively elderly depressed patients, Coffey et al. (1993) first reported volume reduction in the prefrontal cortex. The frontal lobe volume was found to be 7% smaller in inpatients with severe depression (235.88 mL) than in psychiatrically healthy control subjects (254.32 mL). This difference was maintained after adjusting for the effects of age, sex, education, and intracranial size. Kumar et al. (1998) compared 18 patients with late-onset minor depression, 35 patients with late-onset major depression, and 30 nondepressed control subjects. Both elderly groups of patients (minor or major depression) had volume reduction relative to control subjects in prefrontal cortex. Nonetheless, normalized prefrontal lobe volumes showed a significant linear trend with severity of depression, with volumes decreasing with illness severity. These findings suggest that there may be a common neurobiological substrate in diverse forms of late-onset mood disturbance (e.g., minor and major depression). Finally, Kumar et al. (2000) recently examined both prefrontal volume and degree of encephalomalacia in 51 patients with late-life MDD and in 30 nondepressed control subjects. The patient group had both reduced prefrontal volume and greater volume of HI (encephalomalacia). Extent of encephalomalacia correlated significantly among patients with degree of medical comorbidity. However, prefrontal volume reduction and degree of encephalomalacia were not associated, suggesting that these structural abnormalities may represent independent pathological processes in late-life depression.

Using PET functional brain imaging measures in nonelderly samples, Drevets (1998) has shown reduced rCBF and $rCMR_{glu}$ in a specific area of the subgenual prefrontal cortex of patients with unipolar or bipolar depression (also see Chapter 5, this volume). MRI and subsequent neuropathological investigation suggest that there is a pronounced loss of gray matter in this region in both forms of mood disorder. Whether this phenomenon occurs in late-life depression, particularly late-onset MDD, is unknown and of considerable theoretical importance.

In two studies, Sheline and colleagues showed volume reduction in the hippocampus in euthymic women with a history of MDD (Sheline et al. 1999). The volume loss had functional significance, as it was associated with verbal memory deficits. While again this work did not focus on late-life depression, it is of special relevance. The theory guiding this work is that the atrophic effects of stress-related glucocorticoid release during MDD episodes leads to destruction of hippocampal tissue. Indeed, Sheline and colleagues showed that the number of days spent in depressive episodes over patient lifetime is a correlate of hippocampal volume loss, while age alone is not. Given that elderly patients with early-onset depressive illness are likely to have the greatest cumulative lifetime experience of MDD, one should predict that hippocampal volume loss would be most marked in this group. This possibility is under investigation.

Functional Brain Abnormalities

Relatively few studies have used brain imaging techniques to examine functional activity in late-life depression. Furthermore, all studies, whether prior to or following treatment, have examined elderly patients in the resting state. Indeed, across the age span, there has been sparse investigation in major depression of abnormalities in functional activity in the context of affective or cognitive challenge when specific circuits are being activated. Thus, virtually all of our information about functional abnormalities derives from studies of subjects at rest. It is well established in other disorders that challenge conditions can reveal or highlight dysfunctional networks.

Baseline Deficits

There is now an extensive literature documenting abnormalities in resting CBF and CMR in patients in episodes of MDD across the life span. With some notable exceptions (Drevets 1998), most studies report global and/or topographic reductions (most commonly involving prefrontal cortex, caudate nucleus, and cingulate gyrus). Studies in late-life depression (both early and late onset) have generally revealed more profound abnormalities than studies in younger MDD populations. Indeed, the evidence for global reductions in CBF and CMR_{glu} comes almost exclusively from studies of late-life MDD.

Upadhyaya et al. (1990) used HMPAO SPECT to study 18 MDD patients over the age of 66, 14 Alzheimer's disease patients, and 12 normal control subjects. They found a global CBF deficit in the MDD groups (normalized to cerebellum) and regional reductions in frontal, temporal, and parietal regions. Also using HMPAO SPECT, Curran et al. (1993) studied 20 elderly MDD patients (mean age 70) who were receiving medications Their major findings included reduced CBF in frontal and temporal cortex and in anterior cingulate gyrus, thalamus, and caudate nucleus. Bench et al. (1993), using PET, found reduced CBF in dorsolateral prefrontal cortex, angular gyrus, and anterior cingulate gyrus in 40 patients with MDD (mean age 57), half of whom were on medications. Lesser et al. (1994) used both HMPAO SPECT to study regional CBF and the ^{133}Xe inhalation technique to assess global CBF in a sample of 39 medication-free elderly MDD patients in comparison with matched psychiatrically healthy control subjects. Despite being younger than control subjects, the patients had 13.5% reduction in global CBF. Of note, late-onset patients tended to have lower global CBF than early-onset patients. The patients also had topographic reductions in CBF in frontal, temporal, and parietal regions. Two recent HMPAO SPECT studies have further replicated findings of regional CBF reductions in late-life MDD (Awata et al. 1998; Ebmeier et al. 1998). Of note, Ebmeier et al. (1998) also found more extensive perfusion abnormalities in late-onset compared with early-onset patients. In the one study to measure CMR_{glu} in late-life MDD, Kumar et al. (1993) found marked global reductions. The global CMR_{glu} reduction was comparable to that in patients with Alzheimer's disease. In addition, Kumar and colleagues reported regional deficits in prefrontal, temporal, and parietal cortex.

In a series of studies at Columbia University and the New York State Psychiatric Institute, we have examined structural and functional brain abnormalities in late-life MDD. Our first report was on a relatively large sample ($N = 41$) of predominantly elderly (mean age 60.2) inpatients with MDD studied at baseline (eyes closed, at rest) and while free of psychotropic medication, using the ^{133}Xe inhalation planar technique with 32 scintillation detectors (Sackeim et al. 1990). Compared with psychiatrically healthy control subjects ($N = 40$) matched for age, gender, end-tidal pCO_2, blood pressure, and hemoglobin, the depressed group had a marked deficit in global cortical CBF, averaging approximately 12%–14% below normal values. To identify topographic CBF abnormalities, both traditional multivariate techniques and the Scaled Subprofile Model (SSM) were applied. Both SSM and traditional multivariate approaches indicated that depressed patients had CBF reductions in a specific cortical pattern, the *depression profile*. SSM characterized this pattern as involving selective frontal, superior temporal, and anterior parietal regions (see Figure 4–3). The magnitude of this topographic deficit covaried with patient age and severity of depressive symptoms so that older and more severely depressed patients manifested the greatest topographic CBF reduction.

In later work, we contrasted the global and topographic CBF deficits in elderly MDD patients matched to samples of Alzheimer's disease patients and psychiatrically and neurologically healthy control subjects ($N = 30$ per group). Relative to control subjects, the global cortical CBF reduction in MDD patients was of the same magnitude as in Alzheimer's disease patients. As seen in Figure 4–4, this work suggested that the specific topographic abnormality illustrated in Figure 4–3 distinguished depressed patients from both matched control subjects and matched patients with Alzheimer's disease (Sackeim et al. 1993). We have also shown that younger patients with MDD share the prefrontal CBF deficits without the associated reductions in superior temporal and anterior parietal cortex.

Also using the ^{133}Xe inhalation technique, we recently completed a study of 20 elderly depressed outpatients in comparison with 20 matched psychiatrically healthy control subjects (Nobler et al. 2000). Patients averaged 67.8 years of age, met DSM-IV criteria for MDD (unipolar, nonpsychotic; American Psychiatric Association 1994), and at baseline scored at least 18 on the 24-item Hamilton Rating Scale for Depression. They were also free of medical conditions known to compromise CBF measurement

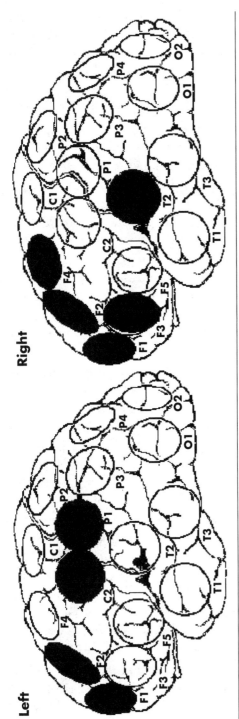

Figure 4–3. Cortical topography found to be abnormal in late-life depression in several studies by the Columbia University group (Nobler et al. 2000; Sackeim et al. 1990, 1993). Thirty-two cortical regions were assessed. Darkened areas reflect regional cerebral blood flow reduction in elderly patients with major depression. The topography reflects abnormalities in prefrontal, superior temporal, and anterior parietal regions.

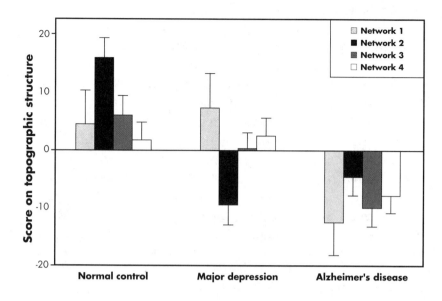

Figure 4–4. The findings of Sackeim et al. (1993). Scores on four topographic patterns for psychiatrically and neurologically healthy control subjects, elderly patients with major depression, and patients with Alzheimer's disease. Depressed patients were abnormal only in the second network, corresponding to the pattern represented in Figure 4–3. The third network presented the abnormality classic in Alzheimer's disease, cerebral blood flow reduction in temporoparietal areas. However, compared to control subjects these patients also showed dysregulation in all four cortical networks. The figure illustrates the specificity of the baseline topographic abnormality in late-life depression.

and were not taking any medication with known effects on CBF. Patients participated in a minimum 14-day psychotropic medication washout, after which baseline CBF assessments were conducted. The depressed sample was contrasted with a normal control group matched for age, sex, and systolic and diastolic blood pressure.

After omnibus testing to establish group differences in regional values, three methods were used to characterize the topographic differences. First, given repeated observations of prefrontal CBF deficits in MDD, an a priori frontal ratio was computed. This corresponded to the mean CBF from 10 frontal detectors (5 per hemisphere) relative to CBF from the remaining 22 posterior detectors.

Second, SSM was applied blind to patient or control status. Each subject was scored for the degree to which each topographic pattern was expressed, as well as for global CBF stripped of topographic contamination. Third, using SSM, scores on the topographic deficit previously obtained in depressed inpatients (Sackeim et al. 1990, 1993), reflecting CBF reductions in selective prefrontal, superior temporal, and anterior parietal regions ("depression profile"), were determined for this new sample. The major findings of this new study were that elderly outpatients in an episode of MDD did not differ from matched psychiatrically healthy control subjects in resting global cortical CBF (unlike the inpatient samples) but had significant topographic reductions in rCBF, principally involving frontal, temporal, and anterior parietal cortical regions. This topographic abnormality was expressed in reduced values for the a priori frontal ratio, in the blind SSM analysis, and when we contrasted scores on a previously obtained depression profile in patients and control subjects.

Overall, the findings from studies of functional brain activity at rest in late-life depression are in broad agreement. In several studies, typically involving inpatients with severe depression, global cortical deficits were observed on the order of 10%–15%. This suggests a marked diminution of synaptic activity across the cortex. There is also concordance in characterizing the cortical areas subject to especially profound functional reduction. These extend broadly across the prefrontal cortex but also involve superior temporal and anterior parietal regions. The cortical deficits in late-life depression may have greater posterior cortical involvement than in younger MDD samples, and the implicated cortical network is known to play a prominent role in motivation and attention.

Treatment and Recovery Effects in Late-Life Depression

Few studies have focused on the changes in functional brain activity that accrue following treatment in late-life depression. A critical question concerns the extent to which CBF and CMR disturbances seen at pretreatment baseline represent state or trait abnormalities. Given the evidence for structural brain abnormalities, it would not be surprising if successful treatment in late-life MDD did not fully reverse baseline functional deficits. Studies of patients before, during, and following treatment will help to answer this question. However, the effects of treatment (whether medications or ECT) on CBF and/or CMR may exert effects independent from those associated with clinical recovery.

Preclinical studies have shown that antidepressant medications, particularly tricyclics, have pronounced effects on capillary permeability, CBF, and CMR, and chronic treatment often results in reduced functional activity in a regionally distributed fashion. In contrast, studies of changes in CBF and CMR following effective pharmacological treatment of MDD in younger adults have yielded inconsistent results. Functional activity has been reported as decreased following treatment, particularly in ventrolateral and orbital frontal cortex. However, several studies have shown no change in at least some baseline cortical abnormalities, while other studies have found at least partial reversal of baseline cortical deficits, particularly in dorsolateral prefrontal cortex, or have found complex patterns of increases and decreases; see Drevets (1998), Sackeim et al. (2000), and Sackeim and Prohovnik (1993) for reviews. None of these studies concentrated on late-life depression. In general, sample sizes have been small, with heterogeneous imaging and treatment methods.

In contrast, findings appear to be more consistent with ECT. With one exception, imaging studies have found decreased CBF or CMR in anterior cortical regions acutely and in the short term following ECT (e.g., Nobler et al. 1994).

Our group has extended the study of abnormalities in CBF in geriatric depression by examining the effects of treatment and clinical response on baseline deficits (Nobler et al. 1994, 2001). Using the ^{133}Xe inhalation technique, rCBF was assessed prior to a course of ECT (pretreatment baseline), 30 minutes before and 50 minutes following a single treatment (acute effects), during the week following the ECT course, and 2 months post-ECT (Nobler et al. 1994). Sixty-eight patients (mean age = 56.8 years) participated across the substudies. Patients were withdrawn from psychotropic medications (other than lorazepam) prior to ECT (mean washout = 19 days). Number of ECT treatments and clinical response were determined by a blind evaluation team. Patients received at least eight treatments before being classified as nonresponders. CBF assessments were made under resting, supine conditions (eyes occluded). Overall, larger acute postictal CBF reductions at the sixth ECT, both globally and in a particular pattern of brain regions, were associated with superior outcome following treatment. Similar patterns were observed during the week following ECT. Global CBF remained reduced (relative to pretreatment baseline) at 2-month follow-up in formerly depressed patients, with strong stability in pretreatment topographic deficit. The findings suggested that baseline CBF abnormalities in MDD were not reversed by successful treatment with ECT. Rather, particularly in responders, ECT led to additional global and topographic CBF reductions, most marked in anterior frontal regions.

In a second study, described earlier (Nobler et al. 2000), 20 elderly outpatients received treatment with antidepressant medication following baseline ^{133}Xe inhalation technique evaluation of rCBF. Eleven patients participated in a double-blind, randomized study of nortriptyline versus sertraline, while the remaining nine patients received nortriptyline in an open fashion. After the patients spent 6–9 weeks on medication, resting rCBF and clinical assessments were repeated. Clinical response was defined as at least a 50% reduction in mean HRSD score from baseline and a final HRSD less than 10. Following the medication trial, 11 patients were nonresponders (9 nortriptyline, 2 sertraline) and 9 were responders (6 nortriptyline, 3 sertraline). There were no differences at baseline or following treatment between responders and nonresponders in age, gender, blood pressure, hemoglobin, or pCO_2 values. Across the sample, there were no changes in these variables across the two time points. Responders averaged an 80.4% decrease (SD = 18.5) in HRSD scores, while nonresponders averaged a 20.8% (SD = 19.5) decrease. Over the treatment course the group as a whole did not change in global CBF. Furthermore, responders and nonresponders did not differ in change in global CBF. In contrast, there was a significant interaction between response status and brain region, indicating that responders and nonresponders differed in the topography of CBF change.

Four topographic patterns were identified by a blind SSM analysis. Responders and nonresponders differed significantly only in the expression of the first pattern. This difference was principally due to responders manifesting CBF reductions in specific prefrontal and anterior temporal regions, a pattern of change not seen in nonresponders. To further test this association, across the sample we correlated scores for change in this topography with depression severity ratings. Greater expression of this pattern of CBF reduction in selective prefrontal and anterior temporal regions following treatment was associated with greater percentage change in HRSD scores from baseline ($r = -0.47$) and lower posttreatment absolute HRSD scores ($r = 0.51$). It did not appear that treatment with nortriptyline or sertraline influenced this relationship. The sample as a whole did not change in expression of the depression profile, and there was no difference between responders and nonresponders in change in this measure. In sum, treatment with antidepressant medications did not result in reversal of the baseline deficit. Instead, pharmacotherapy responders showed further CBF reductions in selective frontal and anterior temporal regions. Furthermore, the magnitude of change in this pattern was correlated with the extent of clinical improvement.

Strikingly, in two independent samples of patients with late-life MDD (Nobler et al. 1994, 2000), successful treatment with either antidepressants or ECT did not reverse baseline CBF reductions. Rather, therapeutic response to both somatic therapies was associated with further deepening of perfusion deficits, suggesting that the CBF abnormalities either represent a trait phenomenon in geriatric depression or that the physiological alterations that result in symptomatic improvement are distinct from the pathophysiology of the illness.

Conclusions

There is growing consensus that the illness of least a subgroup of patients with late-life major depression has a vascular origin.

This view is reinforced by the excess of HI (encephalomalacia) in such patients, suggesting small vessel disease; the association of encephalomalacia with age and cerebrovascular risk factors (e.g., hypertension); the histological evidence indicating that an arteriosclerotic process often is responsible for the HI; and the pathophysiological evidence indicating that encephalomalacia is associated with widespread diminution in cerebral perfusion, limited vascular reserve, and compensatory increases in oxygen extraction. Furthermore, it is evident that, when studied in the depressed state, patients with late-life MDD often have profound disturbances of CBF and CMR. These disturbances characteristically involve prefrontal, superior temporal, and anterior parietal cortical regions but may also reflect global reductions in functional brain activity. Finally, limited study of late-life MDD following response to somatic treatments suggests that baseline abnormalities do not normalize but may in fact become more exaggerated with clinical response. These findings converge on the suggestion that an ischemic disease process, possibly progressive, may be responsible for some manifestations of MDD in late life.

If this is in fact the case, prevention efforts should be directed at developing interventions that limit the incidence of ischemic cerebrovascular disease. Furthermore, treatment of patients with late-life depression should take into account the cerebrovascular action of pharmacological agents. It is conceivable that agents that are acutely effective in suppressing depressive symptoms contribute in the long run to further ischemic damage.

Undoubtedly, there are multiple etiologies to late-life MDD. Indeed, much evidence regarding structural and functional brain abnormalities indicates greater dysfunction in patients with late-onset illness. Commonly, these patients have a low rate of family history of mood disorders, and relations with family history of cerebrovascular or cardiovascular disease have yet to be explored. Especially in patients with late-life MDD and early onset, alternative etiologies are likely at play. These patients also show structural and functional brain abnormalities, but there is a greater likelihood in this group that these deficits reflect the consequences of a lifetime of depressive illness, as opposed to being central etiological factors.

References

Abas MA, Sahakian BJ, Levy R: Neuropsychological deficits and CT scan changes in elderly depressives. Psychol Med 20(3):507–520, 1990

American Psychiatric Association: Diagnostic and Statistical Manual of Mental Disorders, 4th Edition. Washington, DC, American Psychiatric Association, 1994

Andreasen NC, Swayze V 2d, Flaum M, et al: Ventricular abnormalities in affective disorder: clinical and demographic correlates. Am J Psychiatry 147:893–900, 1990

Awad IA, Johnson PC, Spetzler RF, et al: Incidental subcortical lesions identified on magnetic resonance imaging in the elderly, II: postmortem pathological correlations. Stroke 17:1090–1097, 1986a

Awad IA, Modic M, Little JR, et al: Focal parenchymal lesions in transient ischemic attacks: correlation of computed tomography and magnetic resonance imaging. Stroke 17:399–403, 1986b

Awad IA, Spetzler RF, Hodak JA, et al: Incidental subcortical lesions identified on magnetic resonance imaging in the elderly, I: correlation with age and cerebrovascular risk factors. Stroke 17:1084–1089, 1986c

Awad IA, Masaryk T, Magdinec M: Pathogenesis of subcortical hyperintense lesions on magnetic resonance imaging of the brain: observations in patients undergoing controlled therapeutic internal carotid artery occlusion. Stroke 24:1339–1346, 1993

Awata S, Ito H, Konno M, et al: Regional cerebral blood flow abnormalities in late-life depression: relation to refractoriness and chronification. Psychiatry Clin Neurosci 52:97–105, 1998

Aylward EH, Roberts-Twillie JV, Barta PE, et al: Basal ganglia volumes and white matter hyperintensities in patients with bipolar disorder. Am J Psychiatry 151:687–693, 1994

Bench CJ, Friston KJ, Brown RG, et al: Regional cerebral blood flow in depression measured by positron emission tomography: the relationship with clinical dimensions. Psychol Med 23:579–590, 1993

Bird JM, Levy R, Jacoby RJ: Computed tomography in the elderly: changes over time in a normal population. Br J Psychiatry 148:80–85, 1986

Boiten J, Lodder J, Kessels F: Two clinically distinct lacunar infarct entities? A hypothesis. Stroke 24:652–656, 1993

Boone KB, Miller BL, Lesser IM, et al: Neuropsychological correlates of white-matter lesions in healthy elderly subjects: a threshold effect. Arch Neurol 49:549–554, 1992

Breteler MMB, van Amerongen NM, van Swieten JC, et al: Cognitive correlates of ventricular enlargement and cerebral white matter lesions on magnetic resonance imaging: the Rotterdam Study. Stroke 25:1109–1115, 1994a

Breteler MMB, van Swieten JC, Bots ML, et al: Cerebral white matter lesions, vascular risk factors, and cognitive function in a population-based study: the Rotterdam Study. Neurology 44:1246–1252, 1994b

Brown FW, Lewine RJ, Hudgins PA, et al: White matter hyperintensity signals in psychiatric and nonpsychiatric subjects. Am J Psychiatry 149:620–625, 1992

Brown MM, Pelz DM, Hachinski V: Xenon-enhanced CT measurement of cerebral blood flow in cerebrovascular disease (abstract). J Neurol Neurosurg Psychiatry 53:815, 1990

Chimowitz MI, Estes ML, Furlan AJ, et al: Further observations on the pathology of subcortical lesions identified on magnetic resonance imaging. Arch Neurol 49:747–752, 1992

Coffey CE, Figiel GS, Djang WT, et al: Subcortical hyperintensity on magnetic resonance imaging: a comparison of normal and depressed elderly subjects. Am J Psychiatry 147:187–189, 1990

Coffey CE, Weiner RD, Djang WT, et al: Brain anatomic effects of electroconvulsive therapy: a prospective magnetic resonance imaging study. Arch Gen Psychiatry 48:1013–1021, 1991

Coffey CE, Wilkinson WE, Weiner RD, et al: Quantitative cerebral anatomy in depression: a controlled magnetic resonance imaging study. Arch Gen Psychiatry 50:7–16, 1993

Curran SM, Murray CM, Van Beck M, et al: A single photon emission computerised tomography study of regional brain function in elderly patients with major depression and with Alzheimer-type dementia. Br J Psychiatry 163:155–165, 1993

Dahabra S, Ashton CH, Bahrainian M, et al: Structural and functional abnormalities in elderly patients clinically recovered from early and late-onset depression. Biol Psychiatry 44:34–46, 1998

De Reuck J, Decoo D, Strijckmans K, et al: Does the severity of leuko-araiosis contribute to senile dementia? A comparative computerized and positron emission tomographic study. Eur Neurol 32:199–205, 1992

Dolan RJ, Calloway SP, Mann AH: Cerebral ventricular size in depressed subjects. Psychol Med 15:873–878, 1985

Drevets WC: Functional neuroimaging studies of depression: the anatomy of melancholia. Annu Rev Med 49:341–361, 1998

Dupont RM, Jernigan TL, Butters N, et al: Subcortical abnormalities detected in bipolar affective disorder using magnetic resonance imaging. Clinical and neuropsychological significance. Arch Gen Psychiatry 47:55–59, 1990

Dupont RM, Butters N, Schafer K, et al: Diagnostic specificity of focal white matter abnormalities in bipolar and unipolar mood disorder. Biol Psychiatry 38:482–486, 1995

Ebmeier KP, Cavanagh JT, Moffoot AP, et al: Cerebral perfusion correlates of depressed mood. Br J Psychiatry 170:77–81, 1997

Ebmeier KP, Glabus MF, Prentice N, et al: A voxel-based analysis of cerebral perfusion in dementia and depression of old age. Neuroimage 7:199–208, 1998

Elkis H, Friedman L, Wise A, et al: Meta-analyses of studies of ventricular enlargement and cortical sulcal prominence in mood disorders. Comparisons with control subjects or patients with schizophrenia. Arch Gen Psychiatry 52:735–746, 1995

Erkinjuntti T, Gao F, Lee DH, et al: Lack of difference in brain hyperintensities between patients with early Alzheimer's disease and control subjects. Arch Neurol 51:260–268, 1994

Fazekas F, Kleinert R, Offenbacher H, et al: Pathologic correlates of incidental MRI white matter signal hyperintensities. Neurology 43: 1683–1689, 1993

Figiel GS, Krishnan KR, Doraiswamy PM, et al: Subcortical hyperintensities on brain magnetic resonance imaging: a comparison between late age onset and early onset elderly depressed subjects. Neurobiol Aging 12:245–247, 1991

Figiel GS, Krishnan KR, Breitner JC, et al: Radiologic correlates of antidepressant-induced delirium: the possible significance of basal-ganglia lesions. J Neuropsychiatry Clin Neurosci 1(2):188–190, 1989

Figiel GS, Coffey CE, Djang WT, et al: Brain magnetic resonance imaging findings in ECT-induced delirium. J Neuropsychiatry Clin Neurosci 2(1):53–58, 1990

Fujikawa T, Yamawaki S, Touhouda Y: Background factors and clinical symptoms of major depression with silent cerebral infarction. Stroke 25:798–801, 1994

Fujikawa T, Yokota N, Muraoka M, et al: Response of patients with major depression and silent cerebral infarction to antidepressant drug therapy, with emphasis on central nervous system adverse reactions. Stroke 27:2040–2042, 1996

Greenwald BS, Kramer-Ginsberg E, Krishnan KR, et al: MRI signal hyperintensities in geriatric depression. Am J Psychiatry 153:1212–1215, 1996

Greenwald BS, Kramer-Ginsberg E, Krishnan KR, et al: Neuroanatomic localization of magnetic resonance imaging signal hyperintensities in geriatric depression. Stroke 29:613–617, 1998

Hatazawa J, Shimosegawa E, Satoh T, et al: Subcortical hypoperfusion associated with asymptomatic white matter lesions on magnetic resonance imaging. Stroke 28:1944–1947, 1997

Hickie I, Scott E, Mitchell P, et al: Subcortical hyperintensities on magnetic resonance imaging: clinical correlates and prognostic significance in patients with severe depression. Biol Psychiatry 37:151–160, 1995

Hickie I, Scott E, Wilhelm K, et al: Subcortical hyperintensities on magnetic resonance imaging in patients with severe depression: a longitudinal evaluation. Biol Psychiatry 42:367–374, 1997

magnetic resonance imaging and cerebral hemodynamic reserve in carotid occlusive disease. Stroke 28:354–357, 1997

Jacoby RJ, Levy R: Computed tomography in the elderly, III: affective disorder. Br J Psychiatry 136:270–275, 1980

Jenkins M, Malloy P, Salloway S, et al: Memory processes in depressed geriatric patients with and without subcortical hyperintensities on MRI. J Neuroimaging 8:20–26, 1998

Krishnan KR, McDonald WM, Doraiswamy PM, et al: Neuroanatomical substrates of depression in the elderly. Eur Arch Psychiatry Clin Neurosci 243:41–46, 1993

Krishnan KR, Hays JC, Blazer DG: MRI-defined vascular depression. Am J Psychiatry 154:497–501, 1997

Kumar A, Newberg A, Alavi A, et al: Regional cerebral glucose metabolism in late-life depression and Alzheimer disease: a preliminary positron emission tomography study. Proc Natl Acad Sci U S A 90:7019–7023, 1993

Kumar A, Jin Z, Bilker W, et al: Late-onset minor and major depression: early evidence for common neuroanatomical substrates detected by using MRI. Proc Natl Acad Sci U S A 95:7654–7658, 1998

Kumar A, Bilker W, Jin Z, et al: Atrophy and high intensity lesions: complementary neurobiological mechanisms in late-life major depression. Neuropsychopharmacology 22:264–274, 2000

Lebowitz BD, Pearson JL, Schneider LS, et al: Diagnosis and treatment of depression in late life. Consensus statement update. JAMA 278:1186–1190, 1997

Lesser IM, Miller BL, Boone KB, et al: Brain injury and cognitive function in late-onset psychotic depression. J Neuropsychiatry Clin Neurosci 3:33–40, 1991

Lesser IM, Mena I, Boone KB, et al: Reduction of cerebral blood flow in older depressed patients. Arch Gen Psychiatry 51:677–686, 1994

Lesser IM, Boone KB, Mehringer CM, et al: Cognition and white matter hyperintensities in older depressed patients. Am J Psychiatry 153: 1280–1287, 1996

Lopez OL, Becker JT, Rezek D, et al: Neuropsychiatric correlates of cerebral white-matter radiolucencies in probable Alzheimer's disease. Arch Neurol 49(8):828–834, 1992

Meguro K, Hatazawa J, Yamaguchi T, et al: Cerebral circulation and oxygen metabolism associated with subclinical periventricular hyperintensity as shown by magnetic resonance imaging. Ann Neurol 28: 378–383, 1990

Miyao S, Takano A, Teramoto J, et al: Leukoaraiosis in relation to prognosis for patients with lacunar infarction. Stroke 23:1434–1438, 1992

Moody DM, Brown WR, Challa VR, et al: Periventricular venous collagenosis: association with leukoaraiosis. Radiology 194:469–476, 1995

Moore GJ, Bebchuk JM, Wilds IB, et al: Lithium-induced increase in human brain grey matter Lancet 356(9237):1241–1242, 2000

Munoz DG, Hastak SM, Harper B, et al: Pathologic correlates of increased signals of the centrum ovale on magnetic resonance imaging. Arch Neurol 50:492–497, 1993

Nobler MS, Sackeim HA, Prohovnik I, et al: Regional cerebral blood flow in mood disorders, III: effects of treatment and clinical response in depression and mania. Arch Gen Psychiatry 51:884–897, 1994

Nobler MS, Roose SP, Prohovnik I, et al: Regional cerebral blood flow in mood disorders, V: effects of antidepressant medication in late-life depression. Am J Geriatr Psychiatry 8:289–296, 2000

Nobler MS, Oquendo MA, Kegeles LS, et al: Decreased regional brain metabolism after ECT. Am J Psychiatry 158(2):305–308, 2001

O'Brien J, Desmond P, Ames D, et al: A magnetic resonance imaging study of white matter lesions in depression and Alzheimer's disease. Br J Psychiatry 168:477–485, 1996

O'Brien J, Ames D, Chiu E, et al: Severe deep white matter lesions and outcome in elderly patients with major depressive disorder: follow up study. BMJ 317:982–984, 1998

Pearlson GD, Rabins PV, Kim WS, et al: Structural brain CT changes and cognitive deficits in elderly depressives with and without reversible dementia ("pseudodementia"). Psychol Med 19:573–584, 1989

Sackeim HA, Prohovnik I: Brain imaging studies in depressive disorders, in Biology of Depressive Disorders. Edited by Mann JJ, Kupfer D. New York, Plenum, 1993, pp 205–258

Sackeim HA, Steif BL: The neuropsychology of depression and mania, in Depression and Mania. Edited by Georgotas A, Cancro R. New York, Elsevier, 1988, pp 265–289

Sackeim HA, Prohovnik I, Moeller JR, et al: Regional cerebral blood flow in mood disorders, I: comparison of major depressives and normal control subjects at rest. Arch Gen Psychiatry 47:60–70, 1990

Sackeim HA, Prohovnik I, Moeller JR, et al: Regional cerebral blood flow in mood disorders. II: Comparison of major depression and Alzheimer's disease. J Nucl Med 34:1090–1101, 1993

Sackeim HA, Lisanby SH, Nobler MS, et al: MRI hyperintensities and the vascular origins of late life depression, in Progress in Psychiatry. Edited by Andrade C. New York, Oxford University Press, 2000, pp 73–116

Salloway S, Malloy P, Kohn R, et al: MRI and neuropsychological differences in early- and late-life-onset geriatric depression. Neurology 46:1567–1574, 1996

Schlegel S, Maier W, Philipp M, et al: Computed tomography in depression: association between ventricular size and psychopathology. Psychiatry Res 29:221–230, 1989

Sheline YI, Sanghavi M, Mintun MA, et al: Depression duration but not age predicts hippocampal volume loss in medically healthy women with recurrent major depression. J Neurosci 19:5034–5043, 1999

Simpson SW, Jackson A, Baldwin RC, et al: 1997 IPA/Bayer Research Awards in Psychogeriatrics. Subcortical hyperintensities in late-life depression: acute response to treatment and neuropsychological impairment. Int Psychogeriatr 9:257–275, 1997

Swayze VW2, Andreasen NC, Alliger RJ, et al: Structural brain abnormalities in bipolar affective disorder: ventricular enlargement and focal signal hyperintensities. Arch Gen Psychiatry 47:1054–1059, 1990

Tarvonen-Schroder S, Kurki T, Raiha I, et al: Leukoaraiosis and cause of death: a five year follow up. J Neurol Neurosurg Psychiatry 58:586–589, 1995

Thomas AJ, Ferrier IN, Kalaria RN, et al: Elevation in late-life depression of intercellular adhesion molecule-1 expression in the dorsolateral prefrontal cortex. Am J Psychiatry 157:1682–1684, 2000

Upadhyaya AK, Abou-Saleh MT, Wilson K, et al: A study of depression in old age using single-photon emission computerised tomography. Br J Psychiatry Suppl 157:76–81, 1990

JC, van den Hout JH, van Ketel BA, et al: Periventricular
he white matter on magnetic resonance imaging in the elderly: a morphometric correlation with arteriolosclerosis and dilated
perivascular spaces. Brain 114:761–774, 1991

Weinberger DR, Torrey EF, Neophytides AN, et al: Lateral cerebral ventricular enlargement in chronic schizophrenia. Arch Gen Psychiatry
36(7):735–739, 1979

Zubenko GS, Sullivan P, Nelson JP, et al: Brain imaging abnormalities in
mental disorders of late life. Arch Neurol 47:1107–1111, 1990

van Swieten

lesions in

Chapter 5

Neuroimaging Studies of Major Depression

Wayne C. Drevets, M.D.

The application of neuroimaging technology to psychiatric studies is moving understanding of the biology of mood disorders toward an era in which pathophysiology, rather than clinical signs and symptoms, may guide nosology, treatment development, and investigations of etiology. In this process, the knowledge gained from imaging research and from postmortem studies guided by imaging data is catalyzing a paradigm shift in which primary mood disorders are conceptualized as illnesses that involve abnormalities of brain structure as well as of brain function. This chapter reviews the goals and findings of the research program of the author and his collaborators that have contributed to these advances. A review of the neurobiology underlying these imaging findings and their possible relationship to the development of major depressive symptoms is also provided.

The author particularly thanks mentors and/or collaborators Marcus Raichle, M.D., Joseph Price, Ph.D., Tom Videen, Ph.D., Joseph Simpson, M.D., Ph.D., Chet Mathis, Ph.D., David Kupfer, M.D., Ellen Frank, Ph.D., Julie Price, Ph.D., Harold Burton, PhD., Dost Öngür, M.D., Ph.D., Theodore Reich, M.D., Bruce McEwen, Ph.D., Edward Spitznagel, Ph.D., Karen Bell, M.S., and the other co-investigators and research staff who played seminal roles in the training and scientific discussions that led to the research and concepts presented in this chapter.

Overview of the Imaging Research Program

Dependence on a Multidisciplinary Approach

The sheer complexity of clinical neuroscience problems and of the neuroimaging, molecular, neuropathological, and genetic research technologies used to address these problems is most effectively addressed by collaborations involving teams of investigators trained in a variety of disciplines. The studies highlighted below have thus involved psychiatrists, anatomists, neurologists, pharmacologists, chemists, physicists, neurophysiologists, neuroradiologists, geneticists, neuropathologists, cognitive neuroscientists, tracer kineticists, neuroendocrinologists, and statisticians. In addition, the scientists involved have had specialized expertise in particular imaging modalities, enabling us to optimally apply technologies with distinct capabilities and limitations to provide complementary information about pathophysiology.

Major Themes of Neuroimaging Research

Neuroimaging Distinctions Between Major Depressive Subtypes

A broad aim of our studies has been to characterize mood disorder phenotypes based upon neurophysiological, anatomical, neurochemical, and receptor-pharmacological correlates. As a starting point, we employed the state-of-the-art diagnostic assessment reflected in the DSM-series criteria. However, our methods were influenced at Washington University by the iterative, descriptive approaches of Eli Robins, Samuel Guze, George Winokur, and others, who played integral roles in developing the criteria-based syndromes of the DSM classification system. These investigators expected that more innovative clinical-neuroscience approaches to sample selection would ultimately be needed to guide investigations of the pathophysiology and etiology of psychiatric diseases. Consequently, as the early psychiatric imaging literature showed that neuroimaging findings were difficult to replicate across samples selected simply according to DSM-III-R or -IV criteria for major depressive disorder (MDD; American Psychiatric Association 1987, 1994), we began to examine alternative means for selecting subject samples who might be homogenous with respect to pathophysiology.

We initially followed the lead of psychiatric investigators who had demonstrated that specific patterns of family history, clinical course, and psychopathological signs enhanced sensitivity for identifying subject samples more likely to have neuroendocrine, sleep electroencephalogram, and other laboratory abnormalities. We thus examined differences between a) unipolar and bipolar depression, b) familial pure-depressive disease and depression-spectrum disease and sporadic-depressive disease, and c) primary MDD and MDD arising secondary to other conditions. In addition, we distinguished early from late age-at-illness-onset because of the importance of this criterion in the magnetic resonance imaging (MRI) studies of Krishnan et al. (1992, 1993). The importance of such distinctions for the results of imaging studies is reviewed below.

Mood State–Dependent Versus Persistent Abnormalities

A second research aim has been to characterize the time course of imaging abnormalities by scanning mood-disordered subjects in the unmedicated-depressed phase, the treated phase, and the unmedicated-remitted phase of illness. Comparisons across phases allow determination of whether neurophysiological differences between patients with depression and control subjects are evident only during depressive episodes or persist across episodes. They also elucidate neuroimaging correlates of treatment response and predictors of treatment outcome. Such longitudinal imaging studies are being supplemented by cross-sectional studies involving healthy subjects who are at high familial risk for developing mood disorders, in order to distinguish abnormalities that antedate (and may therefore confer vulnerability for) mood disorder onset from those abnormalities that arise as sequelae of chronic or recurrent illness.

Assessing the Relationship Between Functional and Structural Imaging Abnormalities

A research goal that followed from the results of these longitudinal imaging studies has involved characterization of the relationship between functional and structural brain abnormalities in mood disorders. As we discovered focal metabolic deficits that persisted into remission in MDD and bipolar disorder (BD), we initiated in vivo neuromorphometric MRI and postmortem neuropathological investigations of brain structure in the corresponding gray matter regions to determine whether reductions in tissue accounted for our findings. These studies demonstrated that areas of the prefrontal cortex (PFC), amygdala, and striatum display reductions in gray matter volume and associated histopathological changes. Since the physiological measures obtained in these areas using positron emission tomography (PET) are of relatively low spatial resolution, these gray matter abnormalities produce complex relationships between illness severity and observed metabolism. Understanding these relationships has proven essential to the interpretation of antidepressant and mood-stabilizing treatment effects and to the development of neural models of treatment mechanisms.

Emphasis on Anatomical Localization and Neural Circuitry

As anatomical studies have become increasingly specific in delineating subregions of the primate cerebral cortex that are distinct with respect to connectivity and cytoarchitecture, we have attempted to provide localizing information that is as precise as possible, using imaging technology to guide correlations of structure and function. This precision has proven particularly valuable for locating neuroimaging abnormalities to an extent that can guide postmortem neuropathological and receptor-binding studies. Neuroimaging technology is thus applied to delimit both the areas where abnormalities exist and the clinical conditions under which they are evident. Accurate anatomical localization has also proven essential for correlating imaging abnormalities with information regarding anatomical connectivity to guide development of circuitry-based models of mood disorders.

Comparison with Brain Mapping
Studies of Other Emotional States

Finally, to assess the behavioral significance and specificity of functional imaging abnormalities in depression, we are conducting PET and functional MRI (fMRI) brain mapping studies aimed at characterizing normal and pathological emotional states. These studies are elucidating the neurophysiological correlates of anxiety, fear, and sadness and identifying brain areas involved in the inhibition of emotional responses. The results of these studies are interpreted within the context of evidence from lesion analysis and electrophysiological studies in humans and experimental animals regarding the roles these regions play in modulating responses to stressors and emotionally provocative stimuli.

Neurophysiological Imaging
Studies of Major Depression

Interpreting the Biological Significance of
Cerebral Blood Flow (CBF) and
Metabolic Measures in Depression

The interpretation of CBF and metabolic differences between patients with depression and control subjects is complex, requiring thoughtful research design and consideration of data from complementary experimental approaches. Since neural activity, CBF, and glucose metabolism are tightly coupled (Raichle 1987), imaging measures of hemodynamic function and metabolic activity may reflect both the neural processing associated with emotional or cognitive-behavioral symptoms and the pathophysiology underlying vulnerability to mood episodes. Cerebral blood flow and metabolic signals comprise a summation of the chemical processes supporting neural activity, which is dominated by the energy expended during local synaptic transmission (DiRocco et al. 1989; Magistretti et al. 1995; Raichle 1987). Regional elevations of flow and metabolism (i.e., elevated in the experimental condition relative to the control condition) are thus expected to signify increasing afferent synaptic transmission from local or distal structures, while reductions in these measures reflect decreasing afferent transmission (DiRocco et al. 1989; Raichle 1987). Nevertheless, basal CBF and metabolism are affected by alterations in cerebrovascular and neuroreceptor function and in the number of cells and cellular (synaptic) contacts (Chimowitz et al. 1992; Drevets et al. 1999b; Fazekas 1989; Wooten and Collins 1981).

Some of the abnormal elevations in CBF and metabolism found in primary MDD are mood state dependent and are located in regions where CBF also increases in normal and in other pathological emotional states. These differences between patients with depression and control subjects may thus signify areas where physiological activity changes to mediate or adapt to the emotional, behavioral, and cognitive manifestations of the depressive syndrome. Nevertheless, some of these abnormalities are also situated in brain areas where in vivo MRI and postmortem neuropathological studies demonstrate deficits of gray matter volume in primary mood disorders, as reviewed below. The PET data in these regions thus comprise a net summation of the *elevation* of *actual* CBF/metabolism corresponding to activation by the emotive state plus the *reduction* of *apparent* CBF/metabolism caused by the partial volume effect of imaging an area with reduced gray-matter volume using a low-resolution scanner (Links et al. 1996). These competing effects on PET measures give rise to complex relationships between illness severity and observed physiological activity, relationships that can potentially be understood by correcting PET measures for the partial volume effects of the reduction in gray matter volume (Drevets 2000; Mazziotta et al. 1981; Meltzer et al. 1999).

Mood state–dependent *decreases* in CBF and metabolism are also apparent in areas implicated in attentional, visuospatial, and sensory processing during depression (as reviewed in Drevets and Raichle 1998). Interpretation of these findings requires an understanding of the neurophysiological interactions that normally exist across some functional domains within the brain. As humans perform various neuropsychological tasks, PET studies show that CBF increases in brain regions putatively activated to perform the task but concomitantly *decreases* in some other neural systems that appear *nonessential* to task performance (Drevets and Raichle 1998). Such "deactivated" areas are thought to reflect attention-related processes in which signal processing is enhanced by suppressing transmission of unattended information (Drevets et al. 1995a; Posner and Presti 1987).

For example, we demonstrated that during expectation of somatosensory stimulation CBF does not change in the somatosensory cortex representing the skin locus where the stimulus is anticipated, but it decreases in somatosensory cortical regions that represent skin areas *outside* those where stimulation is anticipated (Drevets et al. 1995a). These hemodynamic results putatively reflect the electrophysiological phenomenon of sensory gating, in which neural input to somatosensory cortical neurons is suppressed when the cutaneous receptive field of the recorded cell is not engaged during tactile discrimination behavior and preserved for fields where behaviorally significant stimuli are expected (Chapin and Woodward 1982; Chapman et al. 1991). The reductions in CBF in the cortical areas representing unattended skin sites in our PET study presumably reflected a reduction in afferent synaptic transmission to these areas (Drevets et al. 1995a). PET studies have also shown that similar interactions occur across sensory modalities as well (Drevets and Raichle 1998; Haxby et al. 1994)

The results of PET brain mapping studies further suggest that such cross-modal relationships may exist between areas specialized for emotional versus higher-cognitive functions. In the amygdala and parts of the orbital and ventromedial PFC where flow increases during emotion-related tasks, flow *decreases* while performing attentionally demanding cognitive tasks (Drevets and Raichle 1998; Shulman et al. 1997). Conversely, in dorsolateral PFC and dorsal anterior cingulate areas where flow increases while performing attentionally demanding cognitive tasks, flow *decreases* during some emotional states (Drevets and Raichle 1998; Mayberg et al. 1999).

These reciprocal patterns of neural activity hold intriguing implications for interactions between emotion and cognition. For example, during both the depressed state in MDD subjects and anticipatory anxiety in healthy subjects, CBF decreases in areas of the dorsal anterior cingulate cortex (ACC) that have otherwise been implicated in discriminative attention (Bell et al. 2000; Bench et al. 1992; Drevets and Raichle 1998). This finding may reflect suppression of afferent neural transmission to this area while dysphoric emotions or thoughts are processed. If so, this phenomenon may relate to the subtle impairments of attention associated with depressive episodes. Moreover, because the amygdala and ventral ACC deactivate as the dorsal ACC activates during some types of cognitive processing (Shulman et al. 1997), this phenomenon may also account for why some patients with depression can be distracted from their psychic pain by engagement in attentionally demanding tasks in the workplace.

Critical Assessment of the Psychiatric Imaging Literature

At face value the imaging literature would appear to disagree regarding the specific locations and the direction of neurophysiological abnormalities in mood disorders. However, many inconsistencies across studies can be resolved by considering issues of experimental design and data analysis. Issues related to subject selection, scan acquisition, and image analysis that are particularly relevant for interpreting the author's studies are briefly reviewed here.

Image Acquisition

Our neurophysiological studies of mood disorders have assessed a) glucose metabolism using PET with ^{18}F-fluorodeoxyglucose and b) CBF using PET with $H_2^{15}O$. Perfusion can also be assessed using single photon emission tomography (SPECT) or nontomographic multidetector systems with ^{133}Xe, SPECT with ^{123}I- or ^{99m}Tc-labeled lipophilic agents (e.g., ^{123}I-iodoamphetamine and ^{99m}Tc–hexamethylpropyleneamine oxime [^{99m}Tc-HMPAO]), and, more recently, fMRI. Each method has limitations that must be considered when comparing data across studies using different image acquisition methods.

For example, CBF measures acquired using ^{133}Xe are limited to the gray matter lying within ~2 cm of the scalp (Raichle 1987). Studies employing this tracer are thus unable to examine the amygdala, orbital cortex, and ACC structures emphasized in this chapter. Moreover, assessment of perfusion by ^{123}I-iodoamphetamine and ^{99m}Tc-HMPAO has the limitation that *measured* CBF falls off the line of identity with *actual* CBF at the upper end of the physiological range, so that the sensitivity for detecting areas of *elevated* CBF is reduced. In addition, because CBF is not easily quantitated using ^{123}I-labeled or ^{99m}Te-labeled SPECT tracers, such studies have often normalized perfusion in the target region by perfusion in the cerebellum. However, some PET studies found that flow increases in parts of the cerebellum during depressive and anxiety states (Bench et al. 1992; Drevets and Botteron 1997), so perfusion in other structures may artifactually appear decreased in patients with depression relative to control subjects when normalized to cerebellar flow. It is thus noteworthy that in SPECT studies of MDD, the reported reductions in frontal and temporal perfusion—measured as regional-to-cerebellar ratios—disappear when expressed instead as regional-to-occipital (Philpot et al. 1993) or regional-to-whole cortex (Mayberg et al. 1994) ratios.

Effects of Image Analysis Methods on Statistical Sensitivity

Since the magnitudes of imaging abnormalities in mood disorders have proven to be subtle relative to measurement variability, they have been detectable as statistical differences only between mean measures of ill and control samples. To develop methods for more sensitively comparing image data between patients with depression and control subjects, we have employed a combination of region-of-interest (ROI) and voxel-by-voxel image analysis approaches, which offer different tradeoffs between sensitivity and specificity (Drevets 2000; Poline et al. 1997).

The ROI approach measures PET radiotracer concentration within volumes of interest that are defined in MRI images that have been co-registered to the same subject's PET image. This method provides the greatest sensitivity for detecting abnormalities when the anatomical boundaries of an abnormality are known. However, ROI placement may undersample or dilute abnormalities for which the anatomical boundaries are unknown.

To address this error source, approaches were developed (Drevets et al. 1992; Friston et al. 1991) for comparing images voxel-by-voxel (see Figures 5–1 and 5–2). This requires that the primary tomographs be spatially transformed into standardized stereotaxic space so that image data can be averaged across subjects. A limitation of this method is that current spatial transformation algorithms cannot precisely align the variable, complex structure across brains. To reduce effects of misalignment error, images are blurred ("filtered") prior to analysis (Poline et al. 1997). The reduction of spatial resolution from blurring and the error in overlaying brain structure across subjects decrease sensitivity for detecting abnormalities in small structures or in areas characterized by high anatomical variability (e.g., the orbital cortex).

Voxel-by-voxel analyses may also increase the likelihood of reporting false-positive results, since they require tens or hundreds of thousands of statistical comparisons, increasing the risk that apparent differences will arise by chance alone. This problem can be addressed by correcting P values for the number of independent resolution elements within a search area and constraining the size of the search area (Poline et al. 1997). We have also used an alternative approach in which the significance of apparent differences between groups revealed in voxel-by-voxel analysis is established by targeted ROI analysis of the implicated areas in independent subject samples (Drevets et al. 1992, 1995c, 1997). Unfortunately, few published studies of depression have employed either method for correcting the results of voxel-by-voxel analyses for the number of statistical comparisons, so the literature has been filled with reports of "abnormalities" that likely reflect multiple comparison artifact.

Behavioral State During Scanning

Since functional imaging is sensitive to the neural processing underlying a variety of cognitive-behavioral activities, image data are highly dependent upon the behavioral state during scanning. The major-depressive syndrome comprises a complex state that may differ from the normative state with respect to mood, anxiety, psychomotor activity, sleep deprivation, nutritional state, thought content, attention, and more. Our initial studies

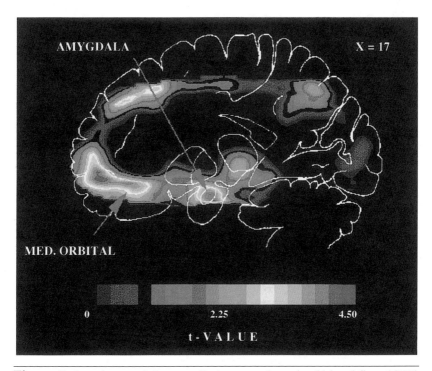

Figure 5–1. Areas of abnormally increased cerebral blood flow (CBF) in familial pure depressive disease. Image shows *t* values produced by a voxel-by-voxel computation of the unpaired *t* statistic for comparison of CBF in depressed and control samples (Drevets et al. 1992). The positive *t* values in this sagittal section at 17 mm left of midline ($x = -17$) show areas of increased CBF in the amygdala and medial orbital cortex in patients with depression relative to control subjects. Abnormal activity in these regions in MDD was confirmed using higher-resolution, glucose-metabolic measures in other studies.
Source.   Modified from Price et al. (1996).

characterized this baseline by scanning subjects in the eyes-closed, at-rest condition because previous literature had shown this state to be stable and reproducible. Interpretation of regional abnormalities thus depended upon subsequent studies in which patients with depression were rescanned in remission, healthy or anxiety disordered subjects were imaged during emotion induction, or patients with depression were studied both at rest and during imposition of specified neuropsychological task states.

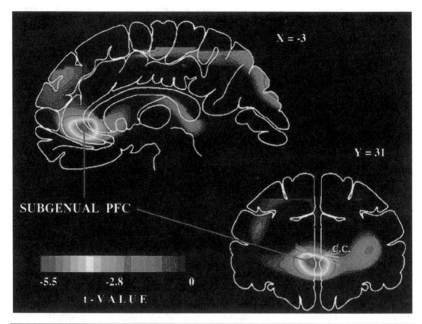

Figure 5–2. Decreased glucose metabolism with depression. Coronal (31 mm anterior to the anterior commissure; $y=31$) and sagittal (3 mm left of midline; $x=-3$) sections show negative voxel t values where glucose metabolism is decreased in patients with depression relative to control subjects (Drevets et al. 1997). The reduction in activity in this region appeared to be accounted for by a corresponding reduction in cortex volume. Although none of these subjects was involved in the study that generated Figure 5–1, the mean metabolism in this independent set of patients with depression was also abnormally *increased* in the amygdala and orbital cortex. Anterior or left is to left. Abbreviation: PFC=prefrontal cortex.
Source. Reprinted with permission from Drevets WC, Price JL, Simpson JR, et al.: "Subgenual Prefrontal Cortex Abnormalities in Mood Disorders." *Nature* 386:824–827, 1997.

While most other laboratories adopted a similar approach, some only imaged depressed subjects performing a specified behavioral task (e.g., receiving mild electrical shocks to the arm or performing the continuous performance task [CPT]; Buchsbaum et al. 1997; Ketter et al. 1999). However, these groups did not examine the effects of affective disease or the depressed state on performance of these tasks and did not compare data acquired in these behavioral states to data acquired in a control condition. Their results have thus been difficult to interpret and cannot be directly compared to those from studies imaging subjects in the eyes-closed, at-rest state.

For example, Shulman et al. (1998) demonstrated that in healthy humans tasks in which visual stimuli are attended to and processed in some way "deactivate" (an effect seen as reductions in CBF) the same amygdala, ventral ACC, lateral orbital cortical, and dorsomedial PFC areas where we observed metabolic abnormalities in patients with depression studied while resting with eyes closed (see below). While some studies that imaged subjects as they performed the CPT obtained findings similar to ours (Cohen et al. 1992), other studies did not (Ketter et al. 1999). It thus remains of scientific interest to determine whether CPT performance differentially deactivates the amygdala, orbital cortex, or dorsomedial PFC in patients with depression versus in control subjects.

Design Issues Related to Sample Selection

Since antidepressant, antianxiety, and antipsychotic drug treatments reportedly decrease CBF and metabolism in frontal, parietal, and temporal lobe regions (as reviewed in Drevets et al. 1999b), we typically image subjects after they have been unmedicated for at least 3 to 4 weeks. Only a minority of other imaging studies of depression have obtained their measures in unmedicated subjects, however. We view this issue as an important source of Type I and Type II errors in the imaging literature, since image data from subjects taking psychotropic drugs often fail to detect the areas of hypermetabolism identified in unmedicated patients with depression, and some report areas of reduced CBF or metabolism not evident in unmedicated samples (as reviewed in Drevets and Botteron 1997).

A Type II error source more difficult to address in imaging studies of mood disorders is the clinical and biological heterogeneity encompassed by the MDD diagnostic criteria. Part of this variability involves clinical differences in severity, chronicity, or signs and symptoms (e.g., psychomotor retardation/agitation), which can be addressed using covariance analysis. However, variability is also introduced by the probability that MDD encompasses a group of disorders that are heterogeneous with respect to etiology and pathophysiology (Drevets and Todd 1997).

Our initial approach to reducing this type of variability has been to select subjects with the familial mood disorder subtypes defined by Winokur (1982). Patients with depression with familial pure depressive disease (FPDD; i.e., primary MDD in an individual who has a first-degree relative with MDD but no first-degree relatives with mania, alcoholism, or antisocial personality disorder) were previously shown to have a higher prevalence of abnormalities of hypothalamic-pituitary-adrenal (HPA)-axis function, platelet [^{3}H]imipramine binding, and sleep electroencephalogram than MDD subjects with sporadic depressive disease (i.e., MDD in an individual lacking mood-disordered relatives) or subjects having first-degree relatives with alcoholism or antisocial personality disorder (depression spectrum disease; Kupfer et al. 1992; Lewis and McChesney 1985; Lewis et al. 1983; Winokur 1982). Patients with depression with FPDD have also been more likely to have elevated CBF and metabolism in the amygdala, orbital cortex, and medial thalamus and decreased metabolism and cortex volume in the subgenual PFC relative to patients with sporadic depressive disease, depression spectrum disease, or depressive syndromes secondary to other conditions (Drevets et al. 1992, 1995b, 1997, 1999b; Hirayasu et al. 1999; Kegeles et al. 1999; Öngür et al. 1998). Nevertheless, alternative means for selecting enriched MDD samples appear to include melancholic subtype criteria or responsiveness to sleep deprivation or phototherapy, which also identify subjects with elevated metabolism in the amygdala and orbital cortex (Cohen et al. 1992; Ebert et al. 1991; Nofzinger et al. 1999; Wu et al. 1992).

Another nosological distinction that appears to influence imaging results is whether a mood disorder has arisen "primary to" other medical or psychiatric conditions or "secondary to" them (i.e., after their onset; Drevets and Todd 1997). For example, the serotonin$_{1A}$ (hydroxytryptamine; 5-HT$_{1A}$) receptor imaging data obtained using PET and the highly selective 5-HT$_{1A}$ receptor radioligand [carbonyl-^{11}C]WAY-100635 (see Figure 5–3; Drevets et al. 1999a; Sargent et al. 2000) converge with the results of in vitro

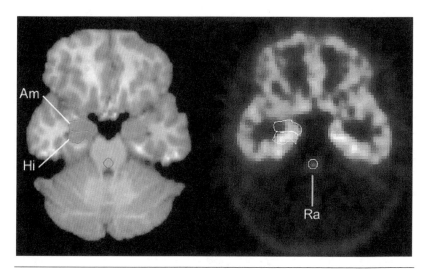

Figure 5–3. Serotonin$_{1A}$ (5-HT$_{1A}$) receptor image. Co-registered magnetic resonance imaging (left) and positron emission tomography (PET; right) sections through the mesiotemporal cortex and midbrain show placement of the hippocampal (Hi), amygdala (Am), and raphe (Ra) regions of interest. The mesiotemporal cortex and anterior cingulate cortex have high 5-HT$_{1A}$ receptor density (hippocampus). The raphe also has high 5-HT$_{1A}$ receptor density and can be visualized in the PET image because the 5-HT$_{1A}$ receptor density in the surrounding mesencephalic and cerebellar tissues is markedly lower. Note the virtual absence of [carbonyl-^{11}C]WAY-100635 uptake in the cerebellum (posterior to the raphe) and white matter, consistent with postmortem measures of 5-HT$_{1A}$ receptor density in humans.
Source. Reprinted with permission from Drevets WC, Frank E, Price JC, et al.: "PET Imaging of Serotonin 1A Receptor Binding in Depression." *Biological Psychiatry* 46(10):1375–1387, 1999.

studies acquired postmortem (Bowen et al. 1989; López et al. 1998) or antemortem (Francis et al. 1989) to indicate that 5-HT$_{1A}$ receptor binding is abnormally decreased in primary MDD and in BD. In contrast, the results of studies of suicide victims who may have had secondary mood disorders or neuropsychiatric conditions other than mood disorders have been highly variable (as reviewed in Drevets et al. 1999b).

Elderly patients with late-onset depression may also comprise a "secondary" mood disorder group with a distinct set of imaging findings. Patients with depression with onset of MDD after age 55 are far more likely than both age-matched, healthy control subjects and age-matched patients with depression with an earlier age at onset to have lacunae in the striatum and large patches of MR signal hyperintensity in T_2-weighted images in the deep and periventricular white matter (Drevets et al. 1999b; Krishnan et al. 1993). Tissue acquired postmortem from brain areas showing these patches reveals arteriosclerosis, white matter necrosis, axon loss, and gliosis within the affected areas proper but not in surrounding tissue where the MR signal appeared normal (Awad et al. 1986; Chimowitz et al. 1992). Functional imaging studies confirm that CBF is decreased in regions where white-matter hyperintensities are evident in MR images (Chimowitz et al. 1992; Fazekas 1989). Patients with late-onset depression also commonly have enlarged cerebral ventricles, widened sulci, and reduced frontal lobe volumes, which may reflect ischemia-induced atrophy (Drevets et al. 1999b). Since cerebrovascular disease alters radiotracer delivery, metabolic activity, and relationships between neuronal activity, oxygen extraction, and CBF (Derdeyn et al. 1998), the functional imaging correlates of late-onset MDD differ fundamentally from those of patients with depression with early or mid-life illness onset (Drevets et al. 1999b). We have consequently excluded elderly subjects and subjects with such MRI abnormalities, and our results are therefore not comparable to those of studies that included elderly patients with depression but failed to exclude subjects with MRI abnormalities.

Functional Anatomical Correlates of Depression

Many of the brain regions where we and others have shown physiological and anatomical abnormalities in MDD and BD have been shown by other types of evidence to participate in the modulation and expression of emotional behavior. Our studies have emphasized assessments of these regions, based upon the expectation that they relate to the core emotional disturbances associated with mood disorders. The following review is, therefore, largely limited to discussion of the neuroimaging data in these regions and of the neurobiological literature relevant to these regions' roles in emotional behavior.

Ventral Anterior Cingulate Gyrus

Subgenual PFC (Subcallosal ACC)

In the ACC ventral to the genu of the corpus callosum (the subgenual PFC), we found that CBF and metabolism are decreased in patients with bipolar depression and in patients with unipolar depression with FPDD relative to those of healthy control subjects (see Figure 5–2; Drevets et al. 1995, 1997). This finding was replicated by Buchsbaum et al. (1997), who termed this area the *rectal gyrus*, and by Kegeles et al. (1999). The metabolic deficit became more pronounced with treatment, so we assessed whether a reduction in tissue volume may account for the reduction in CBF and in metabolism.

We demonstrated a left-lateralized volumetric reduction of the corresponding cortex, initially by MRI-based morphometric measures (Drevets et al. 1997) and later by postmortem neuropathological studies of familial BD and MDD (Öngür et al. 1998). Hirayasu et al. (1999) replicated this MRI finding in a predominantly bipolar sample and extended our results by showing that the gray matter deficit is limited to familial cases and that it is present during the first episode of affective psychosis. In addition, Botteron et al. (in press) found that in twins discordant for MDD the left subgenual PFC volume is decreased in affected twins relative to unaffected co-twins, suggesting that the volumetric deficit may arise following illness onset (Botteron et al. 1999).

Treatment with selective serotonin reuptake inhibitor agents did not alter subgenual PFC volume in MDD (Drevets et al. 1997). In contrast, this volume was significantly larger in BD subjects who had been chronically medicated with lithium or divalproex sodium than in BD subjects who were not medicated with these agents (Drevets et al. 1999). Chronic administration of these mood stabilizers increases expression of the protein Bcl-2 in the frontal cortex, striatum, and mesiotemporal cortex of experimental animals (Manji et al. 1999). Bcl-2 protects against glutamate-mediated excitotoxicity and increases neurite sprouting in vitro, raising the possibility that the difference in subgenual PFC volume in lithium/divalproex-treated BD subjects reflects a neuroprotective/neurotrophic effect of these medications (Manji et al. 1999).

While the *apparent* subgenual PFC metabolism is decreased in PET images from FPDD and BD samples, the actual metabolic activity is seen to be *increased* in patients with depression relative to control subjects once the PET measures are corrected for the partial volume effect of reduced gray-matter volume (Meltzer et al. 1999). When corrected for the reduction in cortex volume, this abnormal elevation of *actual* metabolism appears to fall to normative levels during treatment (Drevets 2000). This reduction in subgenual PFC metabolism in the medicated-remitted phase relative to the unmedicated-depressed phase of MDD has been replicated by Buchsbaum et al. (1997) and Mayberg et al. (1999). The mood state dependency of subgenual PFC activity appears consistent with PET studies showing that flow increases in the subgenual PFC of healthy, nondepressed humans during experimentally induced sadness (Damasio et al. 1998; George et al. 1995; Mayberg et al. 1999).

Pregenual ACC

In the ACC anterior to the genu of the corpus callosum (pregenual ACC) we initially found increased CBF in FPDD (Drevets et al. 1992). This finding has been more difficult to replicate, however, possibly because the pregenual ACC also appears to contain a reduction in cortex and histopathological changes like those identified in the subgenual PFC, potentially giving rise to complex relationships between observed metabolic activity and illness severity (Bell et al. 1999; Cotter et al. 2000). While other laboratories have also reported increased CBF and metabolism in this area during depressive episodes, these data have been inconsistent (Drevets 1999). For example, Mayberg et al. (1997) reported that while metabolism in this area was abnormally increased in patients with depression who subsequently proved responsive to antidepressant drug (AD) treatment, metabolism was decreased in patients with depression who later had poor treatment responses. In contrast, Brody et al. (1999) and Ketter et al. (1999) reported inverse correlations between pregenual ACC metabolism and subsequent antidepressant response in MDD, with lower basal metabolism predicting superior responsiveness to AD treatment. The effects of treatment on pregenual anterior cingulate CBF and metabolism have also differed across studies, with activity decreasing in some but increasing in others following effective treatment (as reviewed in Drevets 1999).

The pregenual ACC more consistently shows areas of elevated hemodynamic activity during anxiety states elicited in healthy or anxiety disordered humans (as reviewed in Drevets and Raichle 1998). Electrical stimulation of this region elicits fear, panic, or a sense of foreboding in humans and vocalization in experimental animals (as reviewed in Price et al. 1996). The relationship between pregenual cingulate activity and the anxiety features associated with MDD thus requires exploration.

Functional Considerations

The subgenual and pregenual ACC share reciprocal anatomical connections with areas implicated in emotional behavior, such as the posterior orbital cortex, amygdala, hypothalamus, accumbens, periaqueductal gray, ventral tegmental area (VTA), raphe, locus coeruleus, and nucleus tractus solitarius (see Figure 5–4; Carmichael and Price 1995; Leichnetz and Astruc 1976). Humans with lesions that include subgenual PFC show abnormal autonomic responses to emotionally provocative stimuli, inability to experience emotion related to concepts, and inability to use information regarding the probability of punishment and reward in guiding social behavior (Damasio et al. 1990). In rats, bilateral or *right*-lateralized lesions of the ventral ACC strip composed of infralimbic cortex, prelimbic cortex (an apparent homologue of primate subgenual PFC), and anterior cingulate cortex (an apparent homologue of primate pregenual ACC) *attenuate* corticosterone secretion, sympathetic autonomic responses, and gastric stress pathology during restraint stress or exposure to fear-conditioned stimuli (Frysztak and Neafsey 1994; Morgan and LeDoux 1995; Sullivan and Gratton 1999). In contrast, *left*-lateralized lesions of this area *increase* sympathetic arousal and corticosterone respons-

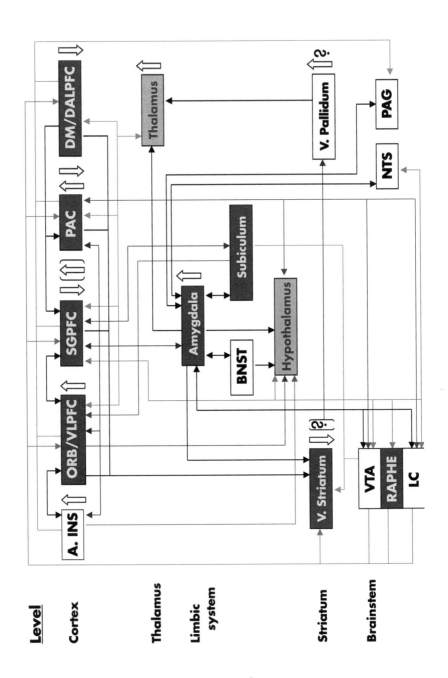

Figure 5–4. Anatomical circuits implicated in familial mood disorders. The regional abnormalities summarized are specifically hypothesized to contribute to the genesis of pathological emotional behavior. Regions shaded in red have neuromorphometric and/or histopathological abnormalities in primary major depressive disorder (MDD) and/or bipolar disorder (BD) (see text). Regions shaded in yellow have not been microscopically examined in mood disorders, but are areas where structural abnormalities are *suspected* based upon the finding of third-ventricle enlargement in children and adults with BD. Open arrows to the right of each region indicate the direction of abnormalities in cerebral blood flow (CBF) and metabolism in patients with depression relative to control subjects; "?" indicates where experimental data await replication. Parenthetical open arrow indicates the direction of metabolic abnormalities after correcting the positron emission tomography (PET) measures for partial volume effects of reduced gray-matter volume; parenthetical question marks indicates where decreased gray matter is suspected as the explanation for reductions in CBF and metabolism, but partial volume-corrected PET results have not been reported. Solid lines indicate *major* anatomical connections between structures; weak projections, such as that from the orbital cortex back to the subiculum (Carmichael and Price 1995), are not included Arrowheads on solid lines indicate the direction of the projecting axons; reciprocal connections have arrowheads at both ends of the line. Affected prefrontal cortex (PFC) areas include the orbital and ventrolateral PFC (ORB/VLPFC), the anterior (agranular) insula (A. Ins), the anterior cingulate gyrus ventral and anterior to the genu of the corpus callosum (subgenual PFC [SGPFC] and pregenual anterior cingulate [PAC], respectively) and the dorsomedial/dorsal anterolateral PFC (DM/DALPFC). The parts of the striatum under consideration are the ventromedial caudate nucleus and nucleus accumbens, which particularly project to the ventral pallidum (Nauta and Domesick 1984). Abbreviations: BNST=bed nucleus of the stria terminalis; NTS=nucleus tractus solitarius; PAG=periaqueductal gray; LC=locus coeruleus; VTA=ventral tegmental area.
Source. Modified from Drevets 2000.

es to restraint stress (Sullivan and Gratton 1999). These data suggest that the right side functions to facilitate expression of visceral responses during emotional processing, while the left subgenual PFC inhibits such responses.

If so, the structural abnormalities of the left ventral ACC in MDD and BD may contribute to the heightened HPA-axis activity and sympathetic autonomic arousal evident in depression (Carney et al. 1988; Dioro et al. 1993; Holsboer 1995; Veith et al. 1994). HPA-axis dysregulation in mood disorders is thought to partly reflect impairment at the level of the limbic system of the negative feedback inhibition on cortisol release (Holsboer 1995; Young et al. 1993). In rats, the ventral ACC contains glucocorticoid receptors that, when stimulated, inhibit stress-induced corticosterone release (Dioro et al. 1993).

Finally, the ventral ACC has been implicated in the evaluation of rewarding stimuli via effects on mesolimbic dopaminergic function. The ventral ACC sends efferent projections to the VTA and the substantia nigra (Leichnetz and Astruc 1976; Price 1999; Sesack and Pickel 1992) and is densely innervated by dopaminergic inputs from the VTA (Crino et al. 1993). In rats, stimulation of medial PFC areas that include prelimbic cortex elicits burst firing patterns from VTA dopaminergic cells and increases dopamine release in the accumbens (Murase et al. 1993; Taber and Fibiger 1993). These phasic, burst firing patterns of dopaminergic neurons participate in encoding information regarding stimuli that predict reward and deviations between such predictions and the actual occurrence of reward (Schultz 1997). Disturbances of the modulatory role the subgenual PFC exerts on VTA neuronal firing activity could thus alter hedonic perception and motivated behavior (Fibiger 1991). In this regard, dysfunction of the subgenual PFC may conceivably relate to switches between depression and mania, as subgenual PFC metabolism (uncorrected for volume) was markedly increased in the manic phase and decreased in the depressed phase of BD (e.g., Drevets et al. 1997).

The Amygdala

We also demonstrated that resting CBF and metabolism are abnormally elevated in the amygdala in FPDD and Type II BD (see

Figure 5–1; Drevets et al. 1992, 1995b, 2000). This abnormality has not been evident in more severe, psychotic BD Type I subjects, primary MDD samples meeting criteria for depression spectrum disease, or secondary MDD samples (Drevets 1995; Drevets et al. 1995c). In subjects who are healthy or have posttraumatic stress disorder (PTSD), CBF has been shown to increase in the amygdala during exposure to emotionally valenced sensory stimuli (Rauch et al. 2000). Nevertheless, abnormalities of *resting* amygdala CBF or metabolism have not been found in PTSD, panic disorder, phobic disorders, obsessive-compulsive disorder (OCD), or schizophrenia, suggesting that this abnormality may be specific to some primary mood disorders (as reviewed in Drevets and Botteron 1997).

Nofzinger et al. (1999) reported that while resting amygdala metabolism is abnormally increased in patients with depression versus control subjects during wakefulness, the normal elevation of metabolism that occurs during rapid eye movement sleep is also greater in patients with depression than in control subjects. These data suggest that the abnormal elevation in amygdala metabolism in major depression is not simply accounted for by an exaggerated subjective response to the stress of scanning.

The magnitude of the elevation of amygdala CBF and metabolism has ranged from 5% to 7% in patients with depression with FPDD relative to healthy control subjects (see Figure 5–5). The actual elevation in amygdala CBF and metabolism would be expected to be ~50% to ~70% in order for PET, which has relatively low spatial resolution, to measure a 5%–7% difference in a structure as small as the amygdala (i.e., comparable in size to an almond; Drevets et al. 1992; Links et al. 1996). Such magnitudes are in the physiological range, as actual CBF increases by 50% in the rat amygdala during exposure to fear-conditioned stimuli (LeDoux et al. 1983).

In some studies, CBF and metabolism in the amygdala have correlated positively with depression severity (Abercrombie et al. 1996; Drevets et al. 1992, 1995b). Consistent with this finding, amygdala metabolism decreases to normative levels during AD treatment that both induces and maintains symptom remission— a result compatible with preclinical evidence that chronic AD

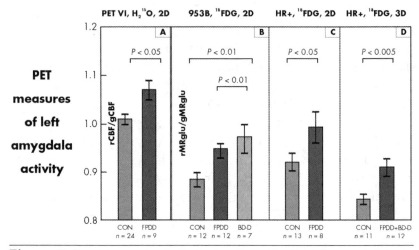

Figure 5–5. Mean physiological activity in the left amygdala in midlife depressed subjects relative to healthy control subjects. Error bars show ±SEM. B, C, and D show the results of three studies obtained with different positron emission tomography (PET) cameras in different laboratories from independent subject samples (as summarized in Drevets et al. 1992, 1995, 1997b, 1999a). *2D* and *3D* refer to image acquisition modes. Abbreviations: rCBF/gCBF = regional-to-global cerebral blood flow ratio; rMRglu/gMRglu = regional-to-global ratio of metabolic rates for glucose; CON = healthy control subjects; FPDD = familial pure depressive disease; BD-D = depressed phase of bipolar disorder.

administration inhibits amygdala function (as reviewed in Drevets 1999). Nevertheless, CBF and metabolism in the left amygdala appeared abnormally increased (albeit to a lesser extent) during the unmedicated, remitted phase of FPDD (Drevets et al. 1992), and AD-medicated, remitted MDD subjects who relapsed in response to serotonin depletion had a higher amygdala metabolism prior to depletion than similar subjects who did not relapse (Bremner et al. 1997). Abnormal amygdala activity may thus be involved in susceptibility to symptom recurrence as well as in episode severity.

The positive correlation between amygdala activity and depression severity may reflect the amygdala's role in organizing multiple aspects of emotional and stress responses. Electrical stimulation of the amygdala in humans increases cortisol secretion and can produce fear, anxiety, dysphoria, and vivid recall of emotionally provocative life events (Brothers 1995; Gloor et al. 1982; Rubin et al. 1966). Amygdala stimulation of the periaqueductal gray (PAG) may conceivably account for depressive signs such as social withdrawal, inactivity, panic attacks, and reduced pain sensitivity, since in experimental animals stimulation of ventrolateral PAG produces behavioral quiescence, social withdrawal, and hypoalgesia, while stimulation of lateral PAG produces sympathetic autonomic arousal, defensive behaviors, and hypoalgesia (as reviewed in Price 1999). Stimulation of amygdala projections to the lateral hypothalamus and locus coeruleus may also increase sympathetic tone, potentially giving rise to the elevated norepinephrine secretion, resting heart rate, and during sleep arousal seen in MDD (Carney et al. 1988; Davis 1992; Veith et al. 1994). Furthermore, the amygdala facilitates stress-related release of corticotropin releasing hormone (CRH; Herman and Cullinan 1997), suggesting a mechanism via which excessive amygdala activity could be involved in inducing the CRH hypersecretion reported in MDD (Feldman et al. 1994; Musselman and Nemeroff 1993). Finally, stimulation of amygdala projections to the ventral striatum arrests goal-directed behavior in experimental animals (Mogenson et al. 1993), suggesting that abnormal amygdala activity may contribute to the reduction in motivated behavior in depression.

Finally, the amygdala participates in the acquisition of emotionally charged or arousing memories (e.g., aversive conditioning) and the evaluation of social stimuli (Büchel et al. 1998; Canli et al. 2000; LaBar et al. 1998; LeDoux 1996; Phelps and Anderson 1997). For example, CBF increases in the amygdala as humans view faces expressing fear or sadness (Blair et al. 1999; Morris et al. 1996), and amygdala lesions impair the ability to recognize fear or sadness in facial expression (Adolphs et al. 1994; Anderson and Phelps 1997) and fear and anger in spoken language (Scott et al. 1997). We found that the pattern of hemodynamic responses to facially expressed emotion is altered in primary mood disorders (Casey et al., in press; Drevets 1999), suggesting the hypothesis that dysfunction involving neural transmission to or within the amygdala alters interpretation of social interactions in depression.

The Orbital and Anterior Insular Cortex

In the posterior orbital cortex, ventrolateral PFC (VLPFC), and anterior (agranular) insula, we and others (e.g., Baxter et al. 1987; Biver et al. 1994; Brody et al. 1999; Cohen et al. 1992; Drevets et al. 1992, 1995c; Ebert et al. 1991) have demonstrated that CBF and metabolism are abnormally increased in *unmedicated* subjects with primary MDD scanned while resting with eyes closed (see Figures 5–1 and 5–4, also Table 3 in Baxter et al. 1987). The elevated activity in these areas in MDD appears mood state dependent, and effective AD treatment results in decreases in CBF and metabolism in the remitted phase relative to the depressed phase (e.g., Brody et al. 1999; Drevets et al. 1992; Drevets 1999; Mayberg et al. 1999; Nobler et al. 1994). Blood flow and metabolism also increase in these areas during induced sadness and anxiety in healthy subjects and induced anxiety and obsessional states in subjects with PTSD, OCD, simple phobia, and panic disorder (Drevets and Raichle 1998).

A complex relationship exists between depression severity and physiological activity in the orbital cortex and VLPFC. While CBF and metabolism increase in these areas in the depressed phase of MDD relative to the remitted phase, the magnitude of these measures correlates inversely with ratings of depressive ideation and severity (Drevets et al. 1992, 1995c). Moreover, while metabolic activity is abnormally increased in these areas in treatment responsive patients with unipolar and bipolar depression, more severely ill or treatment-refractory BD and MDD samples show CBF and metabolic values that do not differ from those of control samples (Drevets 1995).

An inverse relationship between orbital cortex and VLPFC activity and the intensity of emotional behavior is also evident in other conditions. For example, posterior orbital cortex flow increases in OCD subjects and in animal phobic subjects during exposure to phobic stimuli and in healthy subjects during induced sadness (Drevets et al. 1995b; Rauch et al. 1994; Schneider et al. 1995). In these cases, the change in posterior orbital CBF correlated inversely with changes in obsessive thinking, anxiety, and sadness, respectively. In animal phobias, CBF images acquired during repeated exposures to a phobic stimulus revealed that orbital flow progressively increased as subjects habituated to the stimulus, with ΔCBF correlating inversely with changes in heart rate and anxiety (Drevets et al. 1995b).

These data appear consistent with electrophysiological and lesion analysis data showing that parts of the orbital cortex participate in modulating behavioral and visceral responses associated with defensive, fear, and reward-directed behavior as reinforcement contingencies change. Nearly one-half of pyramidal neurons in the orbital cortex alter their firing rates during the delay period between stimulus and response, and this firing activity relates to the presence or absence of reinforcement (Rolls 1995). These cells are thought to play roles in extinguishing unreinforced responses to aversive or appetitive stimuli via their anatomical projections to neurons in the amygdala, striatum, hypothalamus, and other limbic and brainstem structures (Mogenson et al. 1993; Price et al. 1996; Rolls 1995). For example, the orbital cortex and amygdala send direct projections to each other and also have overlapping projections to the striatum, hypothalamus, and PAG through which these structures appear to modulate each other's neural transmission (see Figure 5–4; Carmichael and Price 1995; Garcia et al. 1999; Mogenson et al. 1993; Price 1999). This modulation appears to have behavioral correlation, as defensive behaviors and cardiovascular responses evoked by electrical stimulation of the amygdala are attenuated or ablated by concomitant stimulation of orbital sites, which when stimulated alone have no autonomic effects (Timms 1977). In the depressed phase of FPDD, orbital metabolism is inversely correlated with amygdala metabolism, possibly also reflecting a modulatory influence of orbital activity on amygdala function (Drevets 2000).

Cerebrovascular lesions and tumors involving the frontal lobe increase the risk for developing major depression, although the specific PFC regions where dysfunction confers this risk remain unclear (Mayeux 1982; Starkstein and Robinson 1989). Humans with orbital cortex lesions show impaired performance on tasks requiring application of information related to reward or punishment, perseverate in behavioral strategies that are unreinforced, and exhibit difficulty shifting intellectual strategies in response to changing task demands (Bechara et al. 1998; Rolls 1995). Likewise, monkeys with surgical lesions of the lateral orbital cortex/ VLPFC demonstrate *perseverative interference*, characterized by difficulty in learning to withhold prepotent responses to nonrewarding stimuli as reinforcement contingencies change (Iversen and Mishkin 1970).

Activation of the orbital cortex during depression may reflect endogenous attempts to attenuate emotional expression or interrupt unreinforced aversive thought and emotion. Nevertheless, the neuropathological changes evident in the orbital cortex in primary MDD (Bowen et al. 1989; Rajkowska et al. 1999) raise the possibility that these attempts are ineffective. The abnormalities of monoamine neurotransmitter systems reported in MDD may also impair orbital function. In healthy humans serotonin depletion produces performance deficits on decision-making tasks involving risk/reward probabilities that are similar to those seen in humans with orbital cortex lesions (Rogers et al. 1999), and serotonin-depletion–induced depressive relapse in remitted MDD subjects is associated with metabolic reductions in the orbital cortex and VLPFC (Bremner et al. 1997; the "middle frontal" area of Bremner is the area we have termed VLPFC). Orbital metabolism is also decreased in depressed versus nondepressed subjects with Parkinson's disease, suggesting that dopamine depletion may also impair orbital function (Mayberg et al. 1990; Ring et al. 1994). If neuropathological or monoamine neurotransmitter abnormalities disturb synaptic interactions between the orbital cortex and the amygdala, striatum, hypothalamus, or PAG in mood disorders, emotional behavior may be disinhibited to an extent that pathological emotional responses to stressors and perseverative, nonrewarding/aversive ideation (i.e., obsessive rumination) emerge.

Our finding that CBF and metabolism decrease in the orbital/ insular cortex and VLPFC during effective AD treatment (Drevets et al. 1992, 1997) has been one of the most replicable findings in the literature (as reviewed in Drevets 1999). We have hypothesized that as effective AD treatments directly inhibit pathological limbic activity in areas such as the amygdala, the orbital cortex is no longer activated, as seen by the reduction of metabolism to normal levels. However, two nonpharmacological treatments—

interpersonal therapy and repeated transcranial magnetic stimulation (rTMS)—reportedly *increase* metabolism in the VLPFC and posterior orbital cortex, respectively (Brody et al. 1999; Teneback et al. 1999). Their therapeutic mechanisms may thus depend upon enhancement of PFC mechanisms for modulating emotional expression.

The Dorsomedial/Dorsal Anterolateral Prefrontal Cortex

Another region where dysfunction may impair the ability to modulate emotional responses in mood disorders involves the dorsomedial PFC (DMPFC) and dorsal anterolateral PFC (DALPFC). In a study aimed at replicating and more precisely localizing metabolic deficits reported in these areas by Baxter et al. (1989) and Bench et al. (1992), we iteratively applied ROI and voxel-by-voxel analyses and demonstrated that metabolism was decreased in MDD in the DMPFC (vicinity of dorsal Brodmann areas 32 and rostral 9) and the DALPFC (rostral Brodmann area 9). In the DMPFC, Ring et al. (1994) showed that CBF is also reduced in depressed versus nondepressed patients with Parkinson's disease. In addition, in postmortem studies of the DALPFC, Rajkowska et al. (1999) observed abnormal reductions in the density and size of neurons and glia in MDD, a finding that may relate to the reduction in metabolic activity in this area in PET studies of depression. Consistent with this possibility, the reduction in metabolism in these areas did not normalize during effective AD treatment (Bell et al. 1999), a finding consistent with some but not other PET studies of MDD (reviewed in Drevets et al. 1999b).

Flow increases in the DMPFC in healthy humans as they perform tasks that elicit emotional responses or require emotional evaluations (Dolan et al. 1996; Drevets et al. 1994; Reiman et al. 1997). In healthy humans scanned during anxious anticipation of a mild electrical shock, we observed CBF increases in the DMPFC that correlated inversely with changes in anxiety ratings and heart rate (Drevets et al. 1994), suggesting that this region functions to attenuate emotional expression. In rats, lesions of the area that appears homologous to the primate DMPFC result in exaggerated heart rate responses to fear-conditioned stimuli, and stimulation of these sites attenuates defensive behavior and cardiovascular responses evoked by amygdala stimulation (as reviewed in Frysztak and Neafsey 1994). The DMPFC sends efferent projections to the PAG through which it may modulate cardiovascular responses associated with emotional behavior (Price 1999). Thus, it is conceivable that the metabolic deficits and histological abnormalities found in this area in MDD may result in a disinhibition of some emotional behaviors.

Abnormalities in the Striatum, Thalamus and Other Brain Areas

The orbital cortex, VLPFC, subgenual and pregenual ACC, and amygdala have extensive anatomical connections with the mediodorsal nucleus of the thalamus (MD) and with the ventromedial striatum (Price 1999; Price et al. 1996). In the left medial thalamus, CBF and metabolism are abnormally increased in the depressed phase of FPDD (Drevets et al. 1992, 1995b). In contrast, flow and metabolism are abnormally decreased in the caudate nucleus in MDD (Baxter et al. 1985; Drevets et al. 1992). The volume of the striatum is abnormally decreased in some MRI and postmortem studies of MDD and BD, with the greatest reduction in volume found postmortem in the accumbens area (Baumann et al. 1999; Krishnan et al. 1992). Partial volume effects of this reduction in gray matter may thus partly account for the observed CBF and metabolic reductions in this area in MDD. Nevertheless, depressive relapse induced by acute serotonin depletion in remitted MDD subjects is associated with a reduction in caudate nucleus blood flow, suggesting that dynamic aspects of caudate nucleus function may also be involved in the pathophysiology of major depressive episodes (MDEs) (Smith et al. 1999).

Regional CBF and metabolic abnormalities in other structures have been less consistently replicated. We and others have observed abnormally increased CBF in the posterior cingulate cortex and the medial cerebellum in MDD (Bench et al. 1992; Buchsbaum et al. 1997). Medial cerebellar CBF also increases during experimentally induced anxiety or sadness in healthy or anxiety-disordered subjects (as reviewed in Drevets and Botteron 1997). Some studies have observed reduced CBF and metabolism in lateral temporal and inferior parietal cortical areas in MDD (e.g., Biver et al. 1994; Cohen et al. 1992; Drevets et al. 1992). Some of these areas appear to reflect sensory association cortices, and the significance of reduced activity in these regions in depression remains unclear.

Finally, reductions of CBF and metabolism have been reported in patients with depression versus control subjects in lateral and dorsolateral PFC and in dorsal ACC areas implicated in visuospatial processing and discriminative attention (Bechara et al. 1998; Drevets et al. 1999b; see also review by Drevets and Raichle 1998). These abnormalities appear mood state dependent, reversing during symptom remission (Bench et al. 1995; Mayberg et al. 1999), and initial morphometric and histological assessments have not revealed abnormalities of cortex volume or cell counts in these regions in mood disorders (Bowen et al. 1989; Drevets et al. 1997). The physiological changes in these areas in mood disorders have been linked to the subtle cognitive impairments associated with depression (Dolan et al. 1993). The reductions in physiological activity in these areas may reflect cross-modal suppression of neural transmission of unattended cognitive or behavioral processes, as described above (Drevets and Raichle 1998).

Anatomic Circuits Implicated in MDD

The abnormalities of structure and function in mood disorders implicate limbic-thalamocortical (LTC) circuits involving the amygdala, medial thalamus, orbital and medial PFC, and limbic-cortical-striatal-pallidal-thalamic (LCSPT) circuits, involving the components of the LTC circuit along with related areas of the striatum and pallidum (Drevets et al. 1992). The amygdala and PFC are connected with each other and with MD by excitatory amino acid neurotransmitter projections (Carmichael and Price 1995; Price et al. 1996). Through these connections the amygdala is in a position to activate the PFC both directly and indirectly (through the striatum and pallidum) and to modulate the reciprocal interaction between the PFC and MD (as reviewed in Drevets et al. 1992).

The hypothesized functions of the orbital and medial PFC in modulating emotional and stress responses (discussed above) may be disturbed by dysfunction arising within the PFC itself or within its projection fields in the striatum. Potentially exemplifying this relationship, lesions involving either the PFC or the striatum (e.g., strokes or tumors) and degenerative diseases affecting the striatum (e.g., Parkinson's and Huntington's diseases) are associated with higher rates of secondary major depression than similarly debilitating conditions that spare these regions (Folstein et al. 1991; Mayeux 1982; Starkstein and Robinson 1989). Because these conditions disturb the LCSPT and LTC circuitry in different ways, imbalances within these circuits, rather than overall increased or decreased synaptic activity in a particular structure, may increase the risk for developing a MDE (Drevets et al. 1992).

Nevertheless, some surgical lesions that interrupt projections from the orbital cortex into the striatum can also reduce depressive symptoms. The common mechanism for these neurosurgical interventions for intractable depression (e.g., subcaudate tractotomy, prefrontal/limbic leukectomy; Ballantine 1987; Corsellis and Jack 1973; Knight 1965; Nauta 1973; Newcombe 1975) may be their interruption of amygdala projections into the striatum and ACC. In contrast, the mechanisms for lesions that increase the risk for developing depression may instead involve disinhibition of the amygdala projections into the striatum, ACC, and other limbic structures.

Histopathological Findings in the L-T-C and L-C-S-P-T Circuits

To examine the nature of the reduction in gray matter volume in the subgenual PFC, postmortem studies of the subgenual PFC in MDD and BD were conducted. These studies confirmed the reduction in cortex volume and found that this abnormality was associated with a reduction in glial cells (but no equivalent loss of neurons) and an elevation of neuronal density in subjects in primary MDD and BD (Öngür et al. 1998). Neuropathological findings like those in the subgenual PFC were also made in orbital cortex (Bowen et al. 1989; Rajkowska et al. 1997, 1999), amygdala (Bowley et al. 2000), and pregenual ACC (Cotter et al. 2000). Other areas where volumetric abnormalities are reported in primary mood disorders, such as the ventral striatum and the third ventricle (lined by the medial thalamus and hypothalamus), also implicate structures involved in the LTC and LCSPT circuits, although the histopathological correlates of these abnormalities have not been assessed (Baumann et al. 1999; Drevets and Botteron 1997; Pearlson et al. 1997). In contrast, no differences have been found between midlife or early-onset MDD or between BD subjects and healthy control subjects with respect to the volume of the whole brain, entire PFC, dorsal ACC, and lateral temporal cortex, and the histology of the entorhinal cortex and somatosensory cortex (Bowley et al. 2000; Drevets et al. 1997; Öngür et al. 1998; Pearlson et al. 1997).

While the etiology and time-course of these neuropathological effects are unknown, the histopathology and apparent specificity for areas implicated in the modulation of emotional behavior suggest clues regarding their pathogenesis. The observation that the gray matter volumetric deficit is accompanied by a reduction in glia but no equivalent loss of neurons argues against neurodegenerative hypotheses and instead implies that the neuropil volume is decreased in mood disorders. The neuropil is the moss-like layer of dendritic and axonal fibers that occupies the majority of gray matter volume. The dendritic arborization forming the neuropil can, in some structures, be reversibly "reshaped" in the adult brain by exposure to physiologically elevated concentrations of excitatory amino acid (EAA) neurotransmitters (McEwen 1999). Consistent with the hypothesis that axonal and dendritic arborization is attenuated in the affected regions, the concentrations of various synaptic proteins are decreased in the subgenual and pregenual ACC in BD and MDD, and the mean neuron size is decreased in the pregenual ACC and orbital cortices (Cotter et al. 2000; Eastwood and Harrison, in press; Post et al. 1999).

Dendritic reshaping has been best studied in the hippocampus, where stress-induced elevations in glucocorticoid (e.g., cortisol) concentrations facilitate the EAA-mediated toxicity that produces dendritic atrophy (McEwen 1999; Sapolsky 1996). Stimulation of postsynaptic 5-HT$_{1A}$ receptors protects against this process by maintaining the cytoskeleton (as reviewed in Azmitia 1999). However, the expression of postsynaptic 5-HT$_{1A}$ receptors is down-regulated by stress-induced elevations of adrenal steroid concentrations (López et al. 1998). Primary mood disorders have been associated with impaired negative feedback inhibition of glucocorticoid secretion, reduced serotonergic function, and reduced 5-HT$_{1A}$ receptor binding, suggesting that patients with depression have multiple risk factors that may increase vulnerability to dendritic reshaping (Drevets et al. 2000; Musselman and Nemeroff 1993; Young et al. 1993).

Reduced postsynaptic 5-HT$_{1A}$ receptor function was initially suggested by evidence that patients with major depression have blunted physiological responses to 5-HT$_{1A}$ receptor agonists in vivo and that 5-HT$_{1A}$ receptor and messenger ribonucleic acid concentrations are abnormally decreased in primary MDD postmortem (Bowen et al. 1989; Francis et al. 1993; Lesch et al. 1992; López et al. 1998). Using PET and the selective 5-HT$_{1A}$ receptor radioligand [carbonyl-^{11}C]WAY-100635, we and others demonstrated abnormally decreased 5-HT$_{1A}$ receptor binding potential in the amygdala, hippocampus, raphe, and left orbital cortex in depressed subjects with MDD or BD (see Figure 5–3; Drevets et al. 1999; Sargent et al. 2000). The magnitude of these abnormalities was most prominent in patients with bipolar depression and in patients with unipolar depression who had relatives with bipolar depression.

While elevated cortisol secretion and reduced 5-HT$_{1A}$ receptor function may comprise risk factors for developing reductions in neuropil in widespread brain areas, the targeting of the gray matter volume reductions to specific areas of the LTC and LCSPT circuits (e.g., left, but not right, subgenual PFC; Drevets et al. 1997; Hirayasu et al. 1999) suggests that EAA neurotransmission also plays a role in inducing neuropil alterations in primary mood disorders (McEwen 1999). The finding that during MDE metabolic activity is elevated in the LTC pathway, which is composed of EAA (predominantly glutamatergic) projections, suggests a potential source for chronic glutamate exposure (Drevets et al. 1992). Moreover, glutamate is largely cleared from the extracellular fluid by astrocyte-based transporter sites situated adjacent to synaptic clefts (Magistretti et al. 1995). The glial cell type that has been shown to contribute to the reduction in glia in mood disorders is the astrocyte (Makkos et al. 2000). If the reduction of astroglia found in mood disorders (Rajkowska et al. 2000) impairs the efficiency of glutamate transport, it is conceivable that glutamate concentrations may increase, contributing to the neuropil reduction in limbic regions where glutamate is being actively released. Nevertheless, the only available evidence that glutamate transmission has been elevated in depression is that high-affinity N-methyl-D-aspartate (NMDA) receptors are desensitized in the PFC of suicide victims, suggesting a compensatory response to antemortem exposure to elevated glutamate concentrations (Nowak et al. 1995).

The reductions of gray matter and glia in the subgenual PFC and the elevated metabolism in the LTC circuit have been shown in primary, familial BD or MDD (Drevets et al. 1995; Hirayasu et al. 1999; Öngür et al. 1998) but not in secondary depression or depression spectrum disease. Similarly, depressive subgroups with FPDD or BD have been more likely to have neuroendocrine evidence of elevated limbic HPA-axis activity (e.g., Lewis et al. 1983; Winokur et al. 1982). Finally, the evidence of reduced 5-HT$_{1A}$ receptor binding has been generally limited to studies involving primary mood disorders (Bowen et al. 1989; Drevets et al. 1999a; Francis et al. 1989; López et al. 1998; Sargent et al. 2000), while the 5-HT$_{1A}$ receptor data from suicide victims who may have had secondary mood disorders or neuropsychiatric conditions other than mood disorders have been highly variable (as reviewed in Drevets et al. 1999b). The neuropathological correlates discussed herein may thus be specific to familial mood disorders.

Mood-stabilizing and AD treatments may compensate for impaired glutamate transport, as repeated electroconvulsive shock and chronic AD administration desensitize NMDA-glutamatergic receptors in the rat frontal cortex (Paul et al. 1994), and some anticonvulsant agents that are effective in BD reduce glutamatergic transmission (Sporn and Sachs 1997). Chronic AD and mood stabilizing treatment also appear to increase expression of neurotrophic and neuroprotective factors that may influence the neuromorphometric changes in mood disorders (Duman et al. 1997; Manji et al. 1999). Finally, the putative effects of chronic AD treatment of increasing serotonin transmission, tonically activating postsynaptic 5-HT$_{1A}$ receptors, and enhancing negative feedback inhibition of cortisol release suggest other mechanisms through which such agents may protect against or reverse neuropil reduction (Chaput et al. 1991; Haddjeri et al. 1998; Magarinos et al. 1999; McEwen 1999).

Clinical Implications and Directions for Future Studies

Among the neurobiological questions raised by these imaging and neuropathological data is the critical problem of understanding cause and effect. The extent to which the abnormalities discussed above reflect primary pathology that confers vulnerability to affective disease, as opposed to secondary responses to alterations in behavior, adaptations to chronic illness, or treatment, remains unclear. Future imaging studies of healthy subjects at high familial risk for developing mood disorders, and of the relationships between genetic markers and neuroimaging correlates of illness vulnerability, may elucidate these issues. The combination of neuroimaging and genetic approaches may facilitate discovery of genotypes associated with specific mood-disorder phenotypes (e.g., by delineating trait markers that can guide subject classification in family/genetic studies) and characterize interactions between genetic and environmental factors that produce susceptibility to abnormal mood episodes.

The imaging and neuropathological data reviewed herein indicating that abnormalities of brain structure and function exist in primary mood disorders would also appear to hold profound clinical implications. The persistence of these structural abnormalities into symptom remission potentially provides a neural basis for understanding the recurrent nature of affective disease and the tendency to develop chronicity and treatment resistance following multiple episodes. It also increases the importance of understanding whether the recently discovered neuroprotective and/or neurotrophic effects of some antidepressant and mood-stabilizing treatments can prevent these changes if initiated early in the illness course. If so, the identification of neuroimaging markers for illness vulnerability could then enable development of preventive intervention strategies and identify persons likely to benefit from them.

References

Abercrombie HC, Larson CL, Ward RT, et al: Metabolic rate in the amygdala predicts negative affect and depression severity in depressed patients: an FDG-PET study (abstract). Neuroimage 3:S217, 1996

Adolphs R, Tranel D, Damasio H, et al: Impaired recognition of emotion in facial expressions following bilateral damage to the human amygdala. Nature 372:669–672, 1994

American Psychiatric Association: Diagnostic and Statistical Manual of Mental Disorders, 3rd Edition, Revised. Washington, DC, American Psychiatric Association, 1987

American Psychiatric Association: Diagnostic and Statistical Manual of Mental Disorders, 4th Edition. Washington, DC, American Psychiatric Association, 1994

Anderson AK, Phelps EA: Production of facial emotion following unilateral temporal lobectomy. Society for Neuroscience Abstracts 23:2113, 1997

Awad IA, Johnson PC, Spetzler RJ, et al: Incidental subcortical lesions identified on magnetic resonance imaging in the elderly, II: postmortem pathological correlations. Stroke 17:1090–1097, 1986

Azmitia EC: Serotonin neurons, neuroplasticity, and homeostasis of neural tissue. Neuropsychopharmacology 21(suppl 2):33S–45S, 1999

Ballantine HT Jr, Bouckoms AJ, Thomas EK, et al: Treatment of psychiatric illness by stereotactic cingulotomy. Biol Psychiatry 22:807–819, 1987

Baumann B, Danos P, Krell D, et al: Reduced volume of limbic system-affiliated basal ganglia in mood disorders: preliminary data from a postmortem study. J Neuropsychiatry Clin Neurosci 11(1):71–78, 1999

Baxter LR, Phelps ME, Mazziotta JC, et al: Cerebral metabolic rates for glucose in mood disorders. Arch Gen Psychiatry 42:441–447, 1985

Baxter LR, Phelps ME, Mazziotta JC, et al: Local cerebral glucose metabolic rates in obsessive-compulsive disorder: a comparison with rates in unipolar depression and in normal controls. Arch Gen Psychiatry 44:211–218, 1987

Baxter LR, Schwartz JM, Phelps ME, et al: Reduction of prefrontal cortex glucose metabolism common to three types of depression. Arch Gen Psychiatry 46:243–250, 1989

Bechara A, Damasio H, Tranel D, et al: Dissociation of working memory from decision-making within the human prefrontal cortex. J Neurosci 18(1):428–437, 1998

Bell KA, Kupfer DJ, Drevets WC: Decreased glucose metabolism in the dorsomedial prefrontal cortex in depression (abstract). Biol Psychiatry 45:118S, 1999

Bench CJ, Friston KJ, Brown RG, et al: The anatomy of melancholia: focal abnormalities of cerebral blood flow in major depression. Psychol Med 22:607–615, 1992

Bench CJ, Frackowiak RSJ, Dolan RJ: Changes in regional cerebral blood flow on recovery from depression. Psychol Med 25:247–251, 1995

Biver F, Goldman S, Delvenne V, et al: Frontal and parietal metabolic disturbances in unipolar depression. Biol Psychiatry 36:381–388, 1994

Blair RJR, Morris JS, Frith CD, et al: Neural Responses to sad and angry expressions. Brain 122:883–893, 1999

Botteron KN, Raichle ME, Heath AC, et al: An epidemiological twin study of prefrontal neuromorphometry in early onset depression (abstract). Biol Psychiatry 45:59S, 1999

Bowen DM, Najlerahim A, Procter AW, et al: Circumscribed changes of the cerebral cortex in neuropsychiatric disorders of later life. Proc Natl Acad Sci U S A 86:9504–9508, 1989

Bowley MP, Drevets WC, Öngür D, et al: Glial changes in the amygdala and entorhinal cortex in mood disorders. Society for Neuroscience Abstracts 26:867.10, 2000

Bremner JD, Innis RB, Salomon RM, et al: Positron emission tomography measurement of cerebral metabolic correlates of tryptophan depletion-induced depressive relapse. Arch Gen Psychiatry 54:346–374, 1997

Brody AL, Saxena S, Silverman DHS, Alborzian S, et al: Brain metabolic changes in major depressive disorder from pre- to post-treatment with paroxetine. Psychiatry Research: Neuroimaging 91:127–139, 1999

Brothers L: Neurophysiology of the perception of intentions by primates, in The Cognitive Neurosciences. Edited by Gazzaniga MS. Cambridge, MA, MIT Press, 1995, pp 1107–1116

Büchel C, Morris J, Dolan RJ, et al: Brain systems mediating aversive conditioning: an event related fMRI study. Neuron 20:947–957, 1998

Buchsbaum MS, Wu J, Siegel BV, et al: Effect of sertraline on regional metabolic rate in patients with affective disorder. Biol Psychiatry 41:15–22, 1997

Canli T, Zhao Z, Brewer J, et al: Event-related activation in the human amygdala associates with later memory for individual emotional experience. J Neurosci 20(RC99):1–5, 2000

Carmichael ST, Price JL: Limbic connections of the orbital and medial prefrontal cortex in macaque monkeys, J Comp Neurol 363:615–641, 1995

Carney RM, Rich MW, teVelde A, et al: The relationship between heart rate, heart rate variability and depression in patients with coronary artery disease. J Psychosom Res 32(2):159–164, 1988

Casey BJ, Thomas KM, Eccard CH, et al: Functional responsivity of the amygdala in children with disorders of anxiety and major depression. Biol Psychiatry (in press)

Chapin JK, Woodward DJ: Somatic sensory transmission to the cortex during movement: phasic modulation over the locomotor step cycle. Exp Neurol 78:670–684, 1982

Chapman CE, Ageranioti-Bélanger SA: Discharge properties of neurons in the hand area of primary somatosensory cortex in monkeys in relation to the performance of an active touch tactile discrimination task I: areas 3b and 1. Exp Brain Res 87:319–339, 1991

Chaput Y, deMontigny C, Blier P: Presynaptic and postsynaptic modifications of the serotonin system by long-term administration of antidepressant treatments: an in vivo electrophysiologic study in the rat. Neuropsychopharmacology 5(4):219–229, 1991

Chimowitz MI, Estes ML, Furlan AJ, et al: Further observations on the pathology of subcortical lesions identified on magnetic resonance imaging. Arch Neurol 49:747–752, 1992

Cohen RM, Gross M, Nordahl TE, et al: Preliminary data on the metabolic brain pattern of patients with winter seasonal affective disorder. Arch Gen Psychiatry 49:545–552, 1992

Corsellis J, Jack AB: Neuropathological observations on yttrium implants and on undercutting in the orbito-frontal areas of the brain, in Surgical Approaches in Psychiatry. Edited by Laitinen LV, Livingston KE. Lancaster, England, Medical and Technical Publishing Co, 1973, pp 90–95

Cotter D, Mackay D, Beasley C, et al: Reduced glial density and neuronal volume in major depressive disorder and schizophrenia in the anterior cingulate cortex (abstract). Schizophr Res 41·106, 2000

Crino PB, Morrison JH, Hof PR: Monoaminergic innervation of cingulate cortex, in Neurobiology of Cingulate Cortex and Limbic Thalamus. Edited by Vogt BA, Gabriel M. Boston, MA, Birkhauser, 1993, pp 285–312

Damasio AR, Tranel D, Damasio H: Individuals with sociopathic behavior caused by frontal damage fail to respond autonomically to social stimuli. Behav Brain Res 41:81–94, 1990

Damasio AR, Grabowski TJ, Bechara A, et al: Neural correlates of the experience of emotions. Society for Neuroscience Abstracts 24:258, 1998

Davis M: The role of the amygdala in conditioned fear, in The Amygdala: Neurobiological Aspects of Emotion. Edited by Aggleton JP. New York, Wiley-Liss, 1992, pp 255–230

Derdeyn CP, Yundt KD, Videen TO, et al: Increased oxygen extraction fraction is associated with prior ischemic events in patients with carotid occlusion. Stroke 29(4):754–758, 1998

Dioro D, Viau V, Meaney MJ: The role of the medial prefrontal cortex (cingulate gyrus) in the regulation of hypothalamic-pituitary-adrenal responses to stress. J Neurosci 3(9):3839–3847, 1993

DiRocco RJ, Kageyama GH, Wong-Riley MT: The relationship between CNS metabolism and cytoarchitecture: a review of 14C-deoxyglucose studies with correlation to cytochrome oxidase histochemistry. Comput Med Imag Graph 13:81–92, 1989

Dolan RJ, Bench CJ, Liddle PF: Dorsolateral prefrontal cortex dysfunction in the major psychoses: symptom or disease specificity? J Neurol Neurosurg Psychiatry 56:1290–1294, 1993

Dolan RJ, Fletcher P, Morris J, et al: Neural activation during covert processing of positive emotional expressions. NeuroImage 4:194–200, 1996

Drevets WC: PET and the functional anatomy of major eepression, in Emotion, Memory and Behavior-Study of Human and Nonhuman Primates. Edited by Nakajima T, Ono T. Tokyo, Japan Scientific Societies Press, 1995, pp 43–62

Drevets WC: Prefrontal cortical-amygdala metabolism in major depression, in Advancing from the Ventral Striatum to the Extended Amygdala: Implications for Neuropsychiatry and Drug Abuse. Annals of the New York Academy of Sciences. New York, New York Academy of Sciences, 1999, pp 614–637

Drevets WC: Neuroimaging studies of mood disorders. Biol Psychiatry 48:813–829, 2000

Drevets WC, Botteron K: Neuroimaging in psychiatry, in Adult Psychiatry. Edited by Guze SB. St. Louis, Mosby Press, 1997, pp 53–81

Drevets WC, Raichle ME: Reciprocal suppression of regional cerebral blood flow during emotional versus higher cognitive processes: implications for interactions between emotion and cognition. Cognition and Emotion 12(3):353–385, 1998

Drevets WC, Todd RD: Depression, mania and related disorders, in Adult Psychiatry. Edited by Guze SB. St. Louis, Mosby Press, 1997, pp 99–141

Drevets WC, Videen TO, Price JL, et al: A functional anatomical study of unipolar depression. J Neurosci 12:3628–3641, 1992

Drevets WC, Videen TO, Snyder AZ, et al: Regional cerebral blood flow changes during anticipatory anxiety. Society for Neuroscience Abstracts 20(1):368, 1994

Drevets WC, Burton H, Simpson JR, et al: Blood flow changes in human somatosensory cortex during anticipated stimulation. Nature 373: 249–252, 1995a

Drevets WC, Simpson JR, Raichle ME: Regional blood flow changes in response to phobic anxiety and habituation. J Cereb Blood Flow Metab 15(1):S856, 1995b

Drevets WC, Spitznagel E, Raichle ME: Functional anatomical differences between major depressive subtypes. J Cereb Blood Flow Metab 15(1):S93, 1995c

Drevets WC, Price JL, Simpson JR, et al: Subgenual prefrontal cortex abnormalities in mood disorders. Nature 386:824–827, 1997

Drevets WC, Frank E, Price JC, et al: PET imaging of serotonin 1A receptor binding in depression. Biol Psychiatry 46(10):1375–1387, 1999a

Drevets WC, Gadde K, Krishnan R: Neuroimaging studies of depression, in Neurobiology of Mental Illness. Edited by Charney DS, Nestler EJ, Bunney BJ. New York, Oxford University Press, 1999b, pp 394–418

Duman RS, Heninger GR, Nestler EJ: A molecular and cellular theory of depression. Arch Gen Psychiatry 54:597–606, 1997

Eastwood SL, Harrison PJ: Hippocampal synaptic pathology in schizophrenia, bipolar disorder, and major depression: a study of complexin mRNAs. Molecular Psychiatry 5(4):425–432, 2000

Eastwood SL, Harrison PJ: Synaptic pathology in the anterior cingulate cortex in schizophrenia and mood disorders: a review and western blot study of synaptophysin, GAP-43, and the complexins. Brain Res Bull (in press)

Ebert D, Feistel H, Barocka A: Effects of sleep deprivation on the limbic system and the frontal lobes in affective disorders: a study with Tc-99m-HMPAO SPECT. Psychiatry Research: Neuroimaging 40: 247–251, 1991

Fazekas F: Magnetic resonance signal abnormalities in asymptomatic individuals: their incidence and functional correlates. Eur Neurol 29:164–168, 1989

Feldman S, Conforti N, Itzik A, et al: Differential effects of amygdaloid lesions on CRF-41, ACTH and corticosterone responses following neural stimuli. Brain Res 658:21–26, 1994

Fibiger HC: The dopamine hypotheses of schizophrenia and mood disorders, in The Mesolimbic Dopamine System: From Motivation to Action. Edited by Willner P, Scheel-Kruger J. New York, Wiley, 1991, pp 615–638

Folstein SE, Peyser CE, Starkstein SE, et al: Subcortical triad of Huntington's disease: a model for a neuropathology of depression, dementia, and dyskinesia, in Psychopathology and the Brain. Edited by Carrol BJ, Barrett JE. New York, Raven, 1991, pp 65–75

Francis PT, Poynton A, Lowe SL, et al: Brain amino acid concentrations and Ca2+-dependent release in intractable depression assessed antemortem. Brain Res 494:314–324, 1989

Francis P, Pangalos M, Stephens P, et al: Antemortem measurements of neurotransmission: possible implications for pharmacotherapy of Alzheimer's disease and depression. J Neurol Neurosurg Psychiatry 56:80–84, 1993

Friston KJ, Frith CD, Liddle PF, et al: Comparing functional (PET) images: the assessment of significant change. J Cereb Blood Flow Metab 11:690–699, 1991

Frysztak RJ, Neafsey EJ: The effect of medial frontal cortex lesions on cardiovascular conditioned emotional responses in the rat. Brain Res 643:181–193, 1994

Garcia R, Vouimba R-M, Baudry M, et al: The amygdala modulates prefrontal cortex activity relative to conditioned fear. Nature 402:294–296, 1999

George MS, Ketter TA, Parekh PI, et al: Brain activity during transient sadness and happiness in healthy women. Am. J Psychiatry 152:341–351, 1995

Gloor P, Olivier A, Quesney LF, et al: The role of the limbic system in experiential phenomena of temporal lobe epilepsy. Ann Neurol 12:129–144, 1982

Haddjeri N, Blier P, de Montigny C: Long-term antidepressant treatments result in tonic activation of forebrain 5-HT1A receptors. J Neurosci 18(23):10150–10156, 1998

Haxby JV, Horwitz B, Ungerleider LG, et al: The functional organization of human extrastriate cortex: a PET-rCBF study of selective attention to faces and locations. J Neurosci 14:6336–6353, 1994

Herman JP, Cullinan WE: Neurocircuitry of stress: central control of the hypothalamo-pituitary-adrenocortical axis. Trends Neurosci 20(2):78–84, 1997

Hirayasu Y, Shenton ME, Salisbury DF, et al: Subgenual cingulate cortex volume in first-episode psychosis. Am J Psychiatry 156(7):1091–1093, 1999

Holsboer F: Neuroendocrinology of mood disorders, in Psychopharmacology: The Fourth Generation of Progress. Edited by Bloom FE, Kupfer DJ. New York, Raven, 1995, pp 957–969

Iversen SD, Mishkin M: Perseverative interference in monkeys following selective lesions of the inferior prefrontal convexity. Exp Brain Res 11:376–386, 1970

Kegeles LS, Malone KM, Slifstein M, et al: Response of cortical metabolic deficits to serotonergic challenges in mood disorders (abstract). Biol Psychiatry 45:76S, 1999

Ketter T, Kimbrell TA, Little JT, et al: Differences and commonalties in cerebral function in bipolar compared to unipolar depression. Paper presented at the annual meeting of American College of Neuropsychopharmacology, Acapulco, Mexico, December 1999

Knight G: Stereotactic tractotomy in the surgical treatment of mental illness. J Neurol Neurosurg Psychiatry 28:304–310, 1965

Krishnan KRR, McDonald WM, Escalona PR, et al: Magnetic resonance imaging of the caudate nuclei in depression: preliminary observations. Arch Gen Psychiatry 49:553–557, 1992

Krishnan KRR, McDonald WM, Doraiswamy PM, et al: Neuroanatomical substrates of depression in the elderly. Eur Arch Psychiatry Clin Neurosci 243:41–44, 1993

Kupfer DJ, Targ E, Stack J: Electroencephalographic sleep in unipolar depressive subtypes: support for a biological and familial classification. J Nerv Ment Dis 170(8):494–498, 1992

LaBar KS, Gatenby JC, Gore JC, et al: Human amygdala activation during conditioned fear acquisition and extinction: a mixed trial fMRI study. Neuron 20:937–945, 1998

LeDoux JE: The Emotional Brain. New York, Simon & Schuster, 1996

LeDoux JE, Thompson ME, Iadecola C, et al: Local cerebral blood flow increases during auditory and emotional processing in the conscious rat. Science 221:576–578, 1983

Leichnetz GR, Astruc J: The efferent projections of the medial prefrontal cortex in the squirrel monkey (Saimiri sciureus). Brain Res 109:455–472, 1976

Lesch K: The ipsapirone/5-HT1A receptor challenge in anxiety disorders and depression, in Serotonin 1A Receptors in Depression and Anxiety. Edited by Stahl S, Hesselink JK, Gastpar M, et al. New York, Raven, 1992, pp 135–162

Lewis DA, McChesney C: Tritiated imipramine binding distinguishes among subtypes of depression. Arch Gen Psychiatry 42:485–488, 1985

Lewis DA, Kathol RG, Sherman BM, et al: Differentiation of depressive subtypes by insulin subsensitivity in the recovered phase. Arch Gen Psychiatry 40:167–170, 1983

Links JM, Zubieta JK, Meltzer CC, Stumpf, et al: Influence of spatially heterogenous background activity on "hot object" quantitation in brain emission computed tomography. J Comput Assist Tomogr 20(4): 680–687, 1996

López JF, Chalmers DT, Little KY, et al: Regulation of serotonin1A, glucocorticoid, and mineralocorticoid receptor in rat and human hippocampus: implications for the neurobiology of depression. Biol Psychiatry 43:547–573, 1998

Magarinos AM, Deslandes A, McEwen BS: Effects of antidepressant and benzodiazepine treatments on the dendritic structure of CA3 pyramidal neurons after chronic stress. Eur J Pharmacol 371(2–3):113–122, 1999

Magistretti PJ, Pellerin L, Martin JL: Brain energy metabolism: an integrated cellular perspective, in Psychopharmacology: The Fourth Generation of Progress. Edited by Bloom FE, Kupfer DJ. New York, Raven, 1995, pp 921–932

Makkos Z, Miguel-Hidalgo JJ, Dilley G, et al: GFAP-immunoreactive glia in the prefrontal cortex in schizophrenia and major depression. Society for Neuroscience Abstracts, 2000

Manji HK, Moore GJ, Chen G: Lithium at 50: Have the neuroprotective effects of this unique cation been overlooked? Biol Psychiatry 46:929–940, 1999

Mayberg HS, Starkstein SE, Sadzot B, et al: Selective hypometabolism in the inferior frontal lobe in depressed patients with Parkinson's disease. Ann Neurol 28:57–64, 1990

Mayberg HS, Lewis PJ, Reginald W, et al: Paralimbic hypoperfusion in unipolar depression. J Nucl Med 35:929–934, 1994

Mayberg HS, Brannan SK, Mahurin RK, et al: Cingulate function in depression: a potential predictor of treatment response. Neuroreport 8(4):1057–1061, 1997

Mayberg HS, Liotti M, Brannan SK, et al: Reciprocal limbic-cortical function and negative mood: converging PET findings in depression and normal sadness. Am J Psychiatry 156:675–682, 1999

Mayeux R: Depression and dementia in Parkinson's disease, in Movement Disorders. Edited by Marsden CO, Fahn S. London, Butterworth, 1982, pp 75–95

Mazziotta JC, Phelps ME, Plummer D, Kuhl DE: Quantitation in positron emission computed tomography, V: physical-anatomical effects. J Comput Assist Tomogr 5:734–743, 1981

McEwen BS: Stress and hippocampal plasticity. Annu Rev Neurosci 22:105–122, 1999

Meltzer CC, Kinahan PE, Greer PJ, et al: Comparative evaluation of MR-based partial volume correction schemes for PET. J Nucl Med 40(12):2053–2065, 1999

Mogenson GJ, Brudzynski SM, Wu M, et al: From motivation to action: a review of dopaminergic regulation of limbic → nucleus → accumbens → ventral pallidum → pedunculopontine nucleus circuitries involved in limbic–motor integration, in Limbic Motor Circuits and Neuropsychiatry. Edited by Kalivas PW, Barnes CD. London, CRC Press, 1993, pp 193–236

Morgan MA, LeDoux JE: Differential contribution of dorsal and ventral medial prefrontal cortex to the acquisition and extinction of conditioned fear in rats. Behav Neurosci 109:681–688, 1995

Morris JS, Frith CD, Perrett DI, et al: A differential neural response in the human amygdala to fearful and happy facial expression. Nature 383:812–815, 1996

Murase S, Grenhoff J, Chouvet G, et al: Prefrontal cortex regulates burst firing and transmitter release in rat mesolimbic dopamine neurons. Neurosci Lett 157:53–56, 1993

Musselman DL, Nemeroff CB: The role of corticotropin-releasing factor in the pathophysiology of psychiatric disorders. Psychiatric Annals 23:676–681, 1993

Nauta WJH: Connections of the frontal lobe with the limbic system, in Surgical Approaches in Psychiatry. Edited by Laitinen LV, Livingston KE. Baltimore, University Park Press, 1973, pp 303–314

Nauta WJH, Domesick V: Afferent and efferent relationships of the basal ganglia, in: Function of the Basal Ganglia. CIBA Foundation Symposium 107. London, Pitman Press, 1984, pp 3–29

Newcombe R: The lesion in stereotactic subcaudate tractotomy. Br J Psychiatry 126:478–481, 1975

Nobler MS, Sackeim HA, Prohovnik I, et al: Regional cerebral BF in mood disorders, III: treatment and clinical response. Arch Gen Psychiatry 51:884–897, 1994

Nofzinger EF, Nichols TE, Meltzer CC, et al: Changes in forebrain function from waking to REM sleep in depression: preliminary analyses of [18F]FDG PET studies. Psychiatry Research: Neuroimaging 91:59–78, 1999

Nowak G, Ordway GA, Paul IA: Alterations in the N-methyl-D-aspartate (NMDA) receptor complex in the frontal cortex of suicide victims. Brain Res 675:157–164, 1995

Öngür D, Drevets WC, Price JL: Glial reduction in the subgenual prefrontal cortex in mood disorders. Proc Nat Acad Sci U S A 95:13290–13295, 1998

Paul IA, Nowak G, Layer RT, et al: Adaption of the N-methyl-D-aspartate receptor complex following chronic antidepressant treatments. J Pharmacol Exp Ther 269(1):95–102, 1994

Pearlson GD, Barta PE, Powers RE, et al: Medial and superior temporal gyral volumes and cerebral asymmetry in schizophrenia versus bipolar disorder. Biol Psychiatry 41:1–14, 1997

Phelps EA, Anderson AK: Emotional memory: what does the amygdala do? Curr Biol 7:R311–R314, 1997

Philpot MP, Banaerjee S, Needham-Bennett H, et al: 99mTc-HMPAO single photon emission tomography in late life depression: a pilot study of regional cerebral blood flow at rest and during a verbal fluency test. J Affect Disord 28:233–240, 1993

Poline JB, Holmes A, Worsley K, et al: Making statistical inferences, in Human Brain Function. Edited by Frackowiak R, Friston KJ, Frith CD, et al. London, Academic Press, 1997, pp 85–106

Posner MI, Presti D: Selective attention and cognitive control. Trends Neurosci 10:12–17, 1987

Price JL: Networks within the orbital and medial prefrontal cortex. Neurocase 5:231–241, 1999

Price JL, Carmichael ST, Drevets WC: Networks related to the orbital and medial prefrontal cortex: a substrate for emotional behavior? in Progress in Brain Research: The Emotional Motor System. Edited by Holstege G, Bandler R, Saper CB. Amsterdam, The Netherlands, Elsevier, 1996, pp 523–536

Raichle ME: Circulatory and metabolic correlates of brain function in normal humans, in Handbook of Physiology: The Nervous System V. Edited by Brookhart JM, Mountcastle VB. Bethesda, MD, American Physiological Society, 1987, pp 643–674

Rajkowska G, Selemon LD, Goldman-Rakic PS: Marked glial neuropathology in prefrontal cortex distinguishes bipolar disorder from schizophrenia (abstract). Schizophr Res 24:41, 1997

Rajkowska G, Miguel-Hidalgo JJ, Wei Jinrong, et al: Morphometric evidence for neuronal and glial prefrontal cell pathology in major depression. Biol Psychiatry 45(9):1085–1098, 1999

Rajkowska G: Postmortem studies in mood disorders indicate altered numbers of neurons and glial cells. Biol Psychiatry 48(8):766–777, 2000

Rauch SL, Jenike MA, Alpert NM, et al: Regional cerebral blood flow measured during symptom provocation in obsessive-compulsive disorder using oxygen 15–labeled carbon dioxide and positron emission tomography. Arch Gen Psychiatry 51:62–70, 1994

Rauch SL, Whalen PJ, Shin LM, et al: Exaggerated amygdala response to masked facial stimuli in posttraumatic stress disorder: a functional MRI study. Biol Psychiatry 47:769–776, 2000

Reiman EM, Lane RD, Ahern GL, et al: Neuroanatomical correlates of externally and internally generated human emotion. Am J Psychiatry 154(7):918–925, 1997

Ring HA, Bench CJ, Trimble MR, et al: Depression in Parkinson's disease: a positron emission study. Br J Psychiatry 165:333–339, 1994

Rogers RD, Everitt BJ, Baldacchino A, et al: Dissociable deficits in the decision-making cognition of chronic amphetamine abusers, opiate abusers, patients with focal damage to prefrontal cortex, and tryptophan-deleted normal volunteers: evidence for monoaminergic mechanisms. Neuropsychopharmacology 20:322–339, 1999

Rolls ET: A theory of emotion and consciousness, and its application to understanding the neural basis of emotion, in The Cognitive Neurosciences. Edited by Gazzaniga MS. Cambridge, MA, MIT Press, 1995, pp 1091–1106

Rubin RT, Mandell AJ, Crandall PH: Corticosteroid responses to limbic stimulation in man: localization of stimulus sites. Science 153:767–768, 1966

Sapolsky RM: Stress, glucocorticoids, and damage to the nervous system: the current state of confusion. Stress 1:1–19, 1996

Sargent PA, Kjaer KH, Bench CJ, et al: Brain serotonin1A receptor binding measured by positron emission tomography with [11C]WAY-100635. Arch Gen Psychiatry 57:174–180, 2000

Schneider F, Gur RE, Alav A, et al: Mood effects on limbic blood flow correlate with emotion self-rating: a PET study with oxygen-15 labeled water. Psychiatry Research Neuroimaging 61:265–283, 1995

Schultz W: Dopamine neurons and their role in reward mechanisms. Curr Opin Neurobiol 7:191–197, 1997

Scott SK, Young AW, Calder AJ, et al: Impaired auditory recognition of fear and anger following bilateral amygdala lesions. Nature 385:254–257, 1997

Sesack SR, Pickel VM: Prefrontal cortical efferents in the rat synapse on unlabeled neuronal targets of catecholamine terminals in the nucleus accumbens septi and on dopamine neurons in the ventral tegmental area. J Comp Neurol 320:145–160, 1992

Shulman GL, Corbetta M, Buckner RL, et al: Common blood flow changes across visual tasks, II: decreases in cerebral cortex. J Cogn Neurosci 9(5):647–662, 1997

Smith KA, Morris JS, Friston KJ, et al: Brain mechanisms associated with depressive relapse and associated cognitive impairment following tryptophan depletion. Br J Psychiatry 174:525–529, 1999

Sporn J, Sachs G: The anticonvulsant lamotrigine in treatment-resistant manic-depressive illness. J Clin Psychopharmacol 17(3):185–189, 1997

Starkstein SE, Robinson RG: Affective disorders and cerebral vascular disease. Br J Psychiatry 154:170–182, 1989

Sullivan RM, Gratton A: Lateralized effects of medial prefrontal cortex lesions on neuroendocrine and autonomic stress responses in rats. J Neurosci 19(7):2834–2840, 1999

Taber MT, Fibiger HC: Electrical stimulation of the medial prefrontal cortex increases dopamine release in the striatum. Neuropsychopharmacol 9:271–275, 1993

Teneback CC, Nahas Z, Speer AM, et al: Changes in prefrontal cortex and paralimbic activity in depression following two weeks of daily left prefrontal TMS. J Neuropsychiatry Clin Neurosci 11:426–435, 1999

Timms RJ: Cortical inhibition and facilitation of the defense reaction. J Physiol (Lond) 266:98–99, 1977

Veith RC, Lewis N, Linares OA, et al: Sympathetic nervous system activity in major depression. Arch Gen Psychiatry 51:411–422, 1994

Winokur G: The development and validity of familial subtypes in primary unipolar depression. Pharmacopsychiatry 15:142–146, 1982

Wooten GF, Collins RC: Metabolic effects of unilateral lesion of the substantia nigra. J Neurosci 1:285–291, 1981

Wu J, Gillin C, Buchsbaum MS, et al: Effect of sleep deprivation on brain metabolism of depressed patients. Am J Psychiatry 149:538–543, 1992

Xing G, Zhang LX, Yang S, et al: Increased expression of inducible nitric oxide synthetase and decreased glia fibrillary acidic protein (GFAP) in the post mortem prefrontal cortex of unipolar depressives and schizophrenic individuals. Paper presented at the Annual Meeting of the American College of Neuropsychopharmacology, December 14, 1999

Young EA, Kotun J, Haskett RF, et al: Dissociation between pituitary and adrenal suppression to dexamethasone in depression. Arch Gen Psychiatry 50:395–403, 1993

Afterword

John M. Morihisa, M.D.

The profusion of findings in brain imaging can be scientifically daunting. We often must sift through staggering quantities of data to find a thread of meaning. Indeed, early in the days of brain imaging some scientists criticized the diversity, complexity, and lack of consistency of findings. To some degree this reflected a wide spectrum of approaches, research strategies, and data analysis techniques. Further, there have often been significant differences in equipment and technical approach. In addition, interpretation of data was greatly hampered by the lack of consistent clinical and neuropathological correlations. It might be pointed out that imaging techniques applied to the study of cardiac function have a clarity of meaning and consistency of findings far greater than those seen in brain imaging. However, we have a profoundly superior understanding of the fundamental elements of cardiac activity than of the brain because the heart is a relatively simple mechanism. This has made both the acquisition and the interpretation of cardiac data simple in comparison. The most important reason for the complexity of the findings in brain imaging is the complexity of the brain itself. Furthermore, the challenge of interpreting abnormal findings is greatly exacerbated by our profoundly incomplete understanding of normal brain function. Indeed the failure, thus far, of functional brain imaging to demonstrate clear diagnostic or therapeutic applications in psychiatry is in part due to our need to add to our foundations of knowledge of the brain's neural circuitry. It may also be, as Callicott points out in Chapter 1, that it is more rewarding to use brain imaging to search for specific neuropathology than for pathognomic findings. In this manner we can begin to build a road map of the specific neural networks that are dysfunctional in each disease.

In addition, future investigations will eventually disprove some findings, force reinterpretation of others, and provide a radical realignment of the contextual meaning for yet others. This must give us some pause in our analysis of each study; only carefully and methodically should we add each to our armamentarium of knowledge. Thus, while we must sometimes delay our embrace of scientific data as factual knowledge, this slow and frustrating process should not be a source of pessimism or cynicism. This is clearly a challenging aspect of our field's search for truth, but it is also a normal and necessary part of any scientific endeavor. All scientific investigation can be at times excruciatingly slow in its evolution. Despite the occasional breakthroughs by exceptional minds such as Einstein and Newton, most good science is constructed brick by brick, creating a strong and resilient foundation of understanding upon which future researchers can rely. Indeed, the excitement and joy of science usually consists of making small incremental additions to our knowledge.

Furthermore, as our technology continues to improve and our scientific models become increasingly sophisticated, we will acquire the building blocks of knowledge that will allow us to solve this great mystery—the working of the human mind. Indeed, our myriad techniques of investigation are becoming increasingly powerful due in large part to the innovative minds of researchers who push the technology to its limits with brilliant research paradigms and investigational strategies. We are now on the eve of a new generation of technologies and approaches that hold the promise of fulfilling some of our early expectations. Some of these technologies and strategies have been presented in this volume, such as the compelling work using functional magnetic resonance imaging (fMRI) discussed in Chapters 1, 2, and 3. Perhaps the most encouraging aspect of these papers is the skill with which the technology and the scientific questions are blended in a greater harmony of purpose. This represents a generational improvement over the early brain-imaging studies; scientists have accumulated decades of experience using imaging technology. As this field evolves, we will see an increasingly good fit between the available technology and the often complex questions we wish to pose. Once again the best example of this may be fMRI, which has taken a structural technology that is a reliable cornerstone of medical practice and applied it as an exciting functional research tool with a resolving power unheard of a decade ago.

In this volume the integral connection between the neurosciences and psychiatric research in brain imaging has been demonstrated and its profound influence emphasized. The neurosciences will increasingly drive the direction of brain-imaging investigations. Indeed, research in the neurosciences will shape the very way we conceptualize mental illness. The strongest theme that runs throughout this volume is that research in the basic neurosciences will continue to be one of our most valuable guides in our search for answers to questions such as: what differences in neural network activity characterize major depression?

Various brain imaging techniques and strategies increasingly converge in reporting certain abnormalities. These abnormalities are delineating specific neural networks (such as those involving elements of the prefrontal cortex), which appear to be part of the underlying pathophysiology of mental illnesses. We are thus strongly encouraged to believe that much of the data being generated are incrementally enhancing our foundation of knowledge of how the brain works and how pathological processes affect it. With the inventive strategies developed by these and other scientists, we can begin to see a pattern of meaning to the functioning of the brain, and with this meaning will come greater wisdom.

Index

*Page numbers printed in **boldface** type refer to tables or figures.*

ACC. *See* Anterior cingulate cortex
Adolescents, and depression, 63,
    65-66, 67. *See also* Children
Age at onset, of late-life
    depression, 87-88, 99-100
Aging, and late-life depression, 83
Alzheimer's disease, and late-life
    depression, 86, 92, 102, 107, **109**
Amygdala
    emotion and volume of in
        children, 67
    facial stimuli and social
        phobia, 70-71
    fear conditioning and
        activation of, 69
    neurophysiological imaging
        studies of depression and,
        144-147
Anatomical localization, and
    depression, 126
Animal models
    for DLPFC control of executive
        functions, 33
    for fear conditioning, 61, 62
    for neurophsyiological imaging
        studies of depression, 141,
        150, 151-152
    for working memory in
        schizophrenia, 3, 38

Animal phobias, and posterior
    orbital cortex flow, 148-149
Anterior cingulate cortex (ACC),
    and executive functions
    depression and, 130, 139-144
    obsessive-compulsive
        disorder and, 43-47
    schizophrenia and, 28, 29-32,
        36-43
Anterior insular cortex, and
    depression, 148-151
Antidepressants. *See also* Tricyclic
    antidepressants
    elderly and side effects of, 90
    late-life depression and,
        112-113
    major depression and, 140-141,
        146, 148, 150, 151, 157-158
Antipsychotic medications, and
    movement abnormalities, 6
Anxiety, and neurophysiological
    imaging, 141, 151
Anxiety disorders
    development perspective on
        pediatric, 54, 55-59
    fMRI studies of neural circuits
        in pediatric, 59-74
Arteriosclerosis, and
    encephalomalacia, 92, 93

Attention, and fMRI studies of
neural circuits in children,
64–65, 72–73. *See also*
Executive functions
Attentional set, and executive
control, 33
Auditory hallucinations, and
schizophrenia, 7
Auditory shadowing task, 2
AX continuous performance task
(AX CPT), 39, 41, 43

Baseline deficits, and late-life
depression, 105–110
Bech-Rafaelsen Melancholia
Scale, 101
Behavior. See also Punishment;
Rewards
neuroimaging studies of
depression and state of,
132–135
dispositional tendencies and
associations between adult
and childhood mental
disorders, 59
Bipolar depression. See also
Major depressive disorder
neuroimaging distinctions
and, 125, 156
physiological and anatomical
abnormalities in, 138,
139–140
prefrontal cortex and, 104
Bipolar disorder
fMRI studies of cognitive
deficits in, 10
hyperintensities and, 87
neurophysiological imaging
studies and, **142–143,**
144–145, 148, 152, 154, 155,
156, 157

Blood oxygen level dependent
(BOLD) technique, 67–68
Brain. *See* Amygdala; Anterior
cingulate cortex; Brain
mapping; Cerebral blood
flow; Dorsal prefrontal
cortex; Frontal cortex;
Hippocampus; Neural
circuits; Prefrontal cortex
Brain-behavior relationships, and
cognitive neuroscience, 26
Brain imaging. *See also*
Electroencephalograms;
Functional magnetic
resonance imaging; Labeled-
water positron emission
tomography; Magnetic
resonance imaging;
Neuroimaging research;
Positron emission
tomography; Single-positron
emission computer
tomography
brain mapping in psychiatry
and, 8–13
brain structure and
depression in elderly,
83–114
cognitive neuroscience and,
25–46
critical assessment of
psychiatric literature on,
130–138
development of, 1–3
future of, 171–173
neuroimaging studies of mood
disorders and, 123–159
Brain mapping
dynamic approach to in
psychiatry, 8–13
emotion and, 127

Brain structural morphometry, and late-life depression, 103–105
Brief Psychiatric Rating Scale, 101
Brodmann area, and schizophrenia, 6

Cardiac stress tests, 9, 17
Catechol *O*-methyltransferase (COMT) genotype, and schizophrenia, 9–10, 15
Cerebral blood flow (CBF)
late-life depression and, 95, 96, 105–114, 138
neurophysiological imaging studies of depression and, 127–131, **133, 142–143,** 151, 153
prefrontal cortex function in schizophrenia and, 2–3
Cerebral infarction, and late-life depression, 89
Cerebral vasculature, and schizophrenia, 5
Cerebrovascular disease, and depression, 91–94, 97, 138, 149–150
Children. *See also* Adolescents
developmental perspective on mood and anxiety disorders in, 54, 55–59
fMRI studies of mental disorders in, 53–55, 59–74
structural abnormalities and mood disorders in, **142–143**
Cognitive deficits. *See also* Executive functions; Memory
bipolar disorder and, 10
depression and, 10, 63, 90–91, 101–102
schizophrenia and, 25

Cognitive neurogenetics, 46
Cognitive neuroscience
clinical genetics and, 46
development of, 25–27
executive functions and brain regions, 27–28, 29–47
future of, 46
Cognitive psychology, 25. *See also* Psychological theories
Columbia University, 106–107
Comorbidity, of obsessive-compulsive disorder and neurological disorders, 44
Congruent trial, and ACC function during executive control, 29
Context representation, and executive control, 33
Contextual conditioning, and fear conditioning, 60
Continuous Performance Test, 7
Cortical stress tests, 10
Corticotropin releasing hormone (CRH), 147
Course of illness, and late-life depression, 103
Cybernetic model, of obsessive-compulsive disorder, 44–45

Danger. *See also* Fear
anxiety disorders and, 64
fMRI studies of neural circuits in children and, 60–62
Deep white matter hyperintensity (DWMH), and late-life depression, **86,** 87–88, 89, 90–91, 93
Dendritic reshaping, and hippocampus, 155–156

Depression. *See also* Late-life
   depression; Major depressive
   disorder
   functional anatomical
      correlates of, 138–153
   memory and, 64–65
   neurosurgery and intractable,
      154
   reward-related processes in,
      62–63
Depression profile, 107
Depressive spectrum disease,
   125, 157
Development
   brain circuits and
      psychopathology, 65–66
   developmental dysfunction in
      neural circuits and, 66–74
   model of pediatric mental
      disorders and, 54, 55–59
DLPFC. *See* Dorsal prefrontal
   cortex
Dopamine and dopamine
   system, and orbital cortex,
   150
Dorsal prefrontal cortex (DLPFC)
   ACC function in schizophrenia
      and, 42–43
   executive functions in
      schizophrenia and, 28,
      32–43, 46
   major depressive disorder and,
      94, 151–152
Dorsomedial/dorsal
   anterolateral prefrontal
   cortex (DALPFC), and
   depression, 151–152
DSM-IV diagnostic criteria
   associations between
      disorders in children and
      adults and, 58

for major depressive disorder,
   107, 125
for schizophrenia, 15
Dynamic brain mapping, in
   psychiatry, 8–13

Elderly. *See* Late-life depression
Electroconvulsive therapy (ECT),
   and late-life depression,
   111–112, 113
Electroencephalograms (EEGs)
   error-related negativity (ERN)
      and ACC function, **31**
   genetic studies of
      schizophrenia and, 16
Emotion. *See also* Fear
   brain mapping studies of, 127
   definition of in context, 53
   fMRI studies of neural circuits in
      pediatric mood and anxiety
      disorders and, 59–74
Encephalomalacia
   age at onset of, 87–88
   brain structural abnormalities
      and, 84–87
   cognitive and neurological
      signs of, 90–91
   depressive symptoms and,
      88–89
   etiology of, 91–94
   pathophysiology of, 94–97
   treatment response and
      outcome of, 89–90
Error prevention network, and
   ACC function, 30–31
Error-related negativity (ERN)
   ACC function and, 30–31, 42
   obsessive-compulsive
      disorder and, 45
Etiology, of late-life depression,
   91–94, 114

Evaluative functions. *See also*
 Executive functions
 ACC and performance
  monitoring, 30
 cognitive model of, 28
 frontal cortex and strategic
  processes, **34–35**
Event-related fMRI, and ACC
 function, 42, 45
Excitatory amino acid (EAA)
 neurotransmitters, and
 depression, 155–156
Executive functions. *See also*
 Attention; Cognitive deficits;
 Evaluative functions;
 Memory; Strategic
 functions
 ACC and overcontrol in
  obsessive-compulsive
  disorder, 43–47
 ACC and performance
  monitoring, 29–32
 brain and models of, 27–28
 definition of, 27
 DLPFC and top-down control
  of, 32–36
 schizophrenia and roles of
  ACC and DLPFC in
  impaired, 36–43

Facial expressions, and amygdala
 in social phobia, 70–71
Familial pure depressive disease
 (FPDD), and neurophysio-
 logical imaging studies, 125,
 133, 136, 139, 140, 144–145,
 146, 149, 152, 157
Family studies. *See also* Genetics
 of associations between mental
  disorders in children and
  adults, 57–59

developmental nature of mood
 and anxiety disorders and,
 74
Fear, and fMRI studies of neural
 circuits in children and
 adolescents, 60–62, 68–71. *See
 also* Danger
FLAIR images, and
 encephalomalacia, 84–85
fMRI. *See* Functional magnetic
 resonance imaging
Frontal cortex. *See also* Anterior
 cingulate cortex (ACC)
 reward-related behavior and,
  62
 strategic and evaluative
  processes in, **34–35**
Frontal lobes, and executive
 functions, 28
Functional brain abnormalities,
 and late-life depression,
 105–110
Functional magnetic resonance
 imaging (fMRI)
 advances in brain imaging
  research and, 172, 173
 applications of in psychiatry,
  3–8
 developmental dysfunction in
  neural circuits and, 66–74
 DLPFC and control of
  executive functions, 33–36
 future developments in, 17–18
 genetic studies of
  schizophrenia and, 15–17
 N-back working memory in
  schizophrenia and, 4–5, 39,
  43
 neural circuits in pediatric
  mood and anxiety
  disorders and, 59–66

Functional magnetic resonance
imaging (fMRI) *(continued)*
pathophysiologic studies of
mental disorders in
children and, 53–55

Genetics. *See also* Family
studies
cognitive neuroscience and,
46
developmental perspective on
pediatric mental disorders
and, 56–57
fMRI studies of schizophrenia
and, 15–17
future of brain imaging studies
and, 158
prefrontal cortex function in
schizophrenia and, 9–10
Global Assessment Scale, 101
Glucose. *See* Metabolism,
cerebral

Hamilton Rating Scale for
Anxiety, 101
Hamilton Rating Scale for
Depression (HRSD), 100, 101,
107, 112, 113
Hemodynamics, development
and regulation of peripheral,
74
Heschl's gyrus, and
schizophrenia, 7
Hierarchical model, of
phenomena in mental illness,
58
Hippocampus
dendritic reshaping and,
155–156
major depression and
abnormalities of, 67

Histopathology, and limbic-
cortical-striatal-pallidal-
thalamic and limbic-
thalamocortical circuits,
154–158
Hyperintensities (HI)
bipolar disorder and, 87
late-life depression and, 84, **85,**
86, 91, 93, 95, 96, 114
Hypofrontality, and
schizophrenia, 37

Image acquisition, and
neurophysiological studies
of mood disorders, 130–131
Incongruent trial, and ACC
function during executive
control, 29
Intercellular adhesion molecule-1
(ICAM-1), and late-life
depression, 93–94
Ischemic vascular disease, and
late-life depression, 93–94

Juvenile myoclonic epilepsy, 16

Labeled-water positron emission
tomography ($^{15}O\text{-}H_2O$ PET)
cerebral blood flow in
schizophrenia and, 6
late-life depression and,
94–95
PFC function in schizophrenia
and, 12
working memory in
schizophrenia and, 39
Lacunar infarction, 92
Late-life depression. *See also*
Depression; Major
depressive disorder
age at onset of, 87–88, 99–100

brain structural abnormalities and, 84–87, 97–110
cognitive and neurological signs of, 90–91, 101–102
current understanding of, 83
etiology of, 91–94
pathophysiology of, 94–97, 137–138
severity and nature of symptoms in, 88–89
treatment and outcome of, 89–90, 110–114
Late-Life Depression Clinic, of New York Psychiatric Institute, 84
Leukoaraiosis and leukoencephalopathy. *See* Encephalomalacia
Life course, and childhood origins of chronic mental disorders, 55
Limbic-cortical-striatal-pallidal-thalamic (LCSPT) circuits, and major depressive disorder, 153–158
Limbic system, and fMRI studies of schizophrenia and obsessive-compulsive disorder, 8
Limbic-thalamocortical (LTC) circuits, and major depressive disorder, 153–158
Lithium, and late-life depression, 98
Longitudinal studies
of associations between mental disorders in adults and children, 57–59
developmental nature of mood and anxiety disorders and, 74

of late-life depression, 96–97, 100

Magnetic resonance imaging (MRI). *See also* Functional magnetic resonance imaging (fMRI)
late-life depression and, 85–87
structural studies of pediatric mood and anxiety disorders and, 66–67
Major depressive disorder (MDD). *See also* Bipolar depression; Depression; Late-life depression; Mood disorders; Unipolar depression
adolescence and increase of, 65–66
anatomic circuits and, 153–158
fMRI studies of cognitive deficits in, 10
limbic-thalamocortical (LTC) circuits and, 153–158
neuroimaging distinctions between subtypes of, 124–125
neurophysiological imaging studies of, 127–138
prefrontal volumes in children and adolescents with, 67
Medial cerebellum, and major depressive disorder, 152–153
Memory. *See also* Cognitive deficits; Executive functions; Working memory
amygdala and, 147
declarative forms of, 73
depression and, 64–65
fMRI studies of neural circuits in children and, 64, 72–73

Metabolism, cerebral (CMR)
late-life depression and, 105–114
neurophysiological imaging
studies of major
depression and, 127–130,
134, 142–143, 153
Met-Met individuals, and
schizophrenia, 10
Microatheromatosis, and
encephalomalacia, 92
Mini-Mental State Exam, 91, 102
Monoamine oxidase inhibitors
(MAOIs), and late-life
depression, 98
Mood disorders. *See also* Major
depressive disorder
developmental perspective on
pediatric, 54, 55–59
fMRI studies of neural circuits
in pediatric, 59–74
neuroimaging technology and
paradigm shift in concept
of, 123
Mood state-dependent
depression, 125
Motor abnormalities, and fMRI
studies of schizophrenia, 6
Multi-infarct dementia, and
encephalomalacia, 87

N-acetylaspartate (NAA)
major depressive disorder and,
157
schizophrenia and, 11–13, 16–17
N-back working memory, and
schizophrenia, 4–5, 39, **40,** 43
Neural circuits. *See also*
Neurological disorders
fMRI studies of pediatric
mood and anxiety
disorders, 59–74

neuroimaging research on
depression and, 126
Neuroimaging research
anatomic circuits in major
depressive disorder and,
153–158
clinical implications of, 158
functional anatomical
correlates of depression
and, 138–153
future of, 158–159
major themes of, 124–127
multidisciplinary approach in,
124
neurophysiological imaging
studies of major
depression and, 127–138
paradigm shift in concept of
mood disorders and, 123
Neuroleptics, and late-life
depression, 98
Neurological disorders. *See also*
Neural circuits;
Neurophysiological imaging;
Neurosurgery
comorbidity with obsessive-
compulsive disorder, 44
signs of late-life depression
and, 90–91
Neuronal density, and
schizophrenia, 1, 6
Neurophysiological imaging,
and studies of major
depression, 127–138. *See also*
Neurological disorders
Neurosurgery
intractable depression and, 154
obsessive-compulsive
disorder and, 44
New York Psychiatric Institute,
84, 106–107

Nortriptyline, and late-life depression, 112–113

Obsessive-compulsive disorder (OCD)
amygdala volume and, 67
fMRI studies of limbic system and, 8
overcontrol and performance monitoring in, 43–47
posterior orbital cortex flow and, 148–149
Orbital insular cortex, and depression, 148–151
Outcome, of treatment in late-life depression, 89–90
Overcontrol, and performance monitoring in obsessive-compulsive disorder, 43–47

Panic disorder, and children, 57
Parkinson's disease, 150, 151
Partial errors, and ERNs, 30
Pathophysiology, of encephalomalacia, 94–97
Patient motion, and fMRI studies, 4
Performance monitoring
ACC function in schizophrenia and, 29–32, 41–43
cognitive models of executive function and, 28
overcontrol and role of ACC in obsessive-compulsive disorder and, 43–47
Periaqueductal gray (PAG), and depression, 147
Periodic task design, and stimulus-correlated motion, 5

Periventricular hyperintensities (PVHs), and late-life depression, 84, **85**, 86, 93, 95
Perseverative interference, and learning, 150
Persistent abnormalities, and depression, 125
PFC. *See* Prefrontal cortex
Phenomenology, of late-life depression, 100–101
Phobias. *See* Animal phobias; Social phobia
Photic stimulation, and schizophrenia, 5–6
Physiology, and cognitive neuroscience, 25. *See also* Neurophysiological imaging
Plasticity, and development, 73–74
Positive symptoms, of schizophrenia, 7
Positron emission tomography (PET). *See also* Labeled-water positron emission tomography
cerebral blood flow and metabolism in depression and, 128–129, **142–143**
fear-related processes in children and adolescents and, 68–69
frontal cortex and symptoms of obsessive-compulsive disorder, 44
late-life depression and, 94–95, 106
prefrontal cortex and unipolar and bipolar depression, 104
subgenual PFC metabolism in depression and, 140

Posttraumatic stress disorder (PTSD), and cerebral blood flow in amygdala, 145

Prefrontal cortex (PFC). *See also* Dorsal prefrontal cortex; Ventral prefrontal cortex
fMRI studies of schizophrenia and, 7–8, 10–13, 17
major depressive disorder and, 139–140, 148–152
reduced function in schizophrenia and, 2–3, 9–10

Pregenual ACC, and neurophysiological imaging studies of depression, 140–144

Prevention, of late-life depression, 114

Pseudodementia, 102

Psychiatry. *See also* Anxiety disorders; Bipolar disorder; Depression; Mood disorders; Obsessive-compulsive disorder; Panic disorder; Posttraumatic stress disorder; Schizophrenia; Social phobia
applications of fMRI in, 3–8
critical assessment of literature on brain imaging and, 130–138
dynamic approach to brain mapping in, 8–13

Psychological theories, of obsessive-compulsive disorder, 43. *See also* Cognitive psychology

Puberty, and neural or cognitive development, 65–66

Punishment, definition of in context, 53. *See also* Rewards

Rating for Emotional Blunting, 101

Recovery efforts, and late-life depression, 110–114

Rectal gyrus. *See* Subgenual PFC

Region-of-interest (ROI) image analysis, 131–132

Relative risk statistic, and genetic studies of schizophrenia, 16

Repeated transcranial magnetic stimulation (rTMS), 151

Research. *See* Neuroimaging research; Research design

Research design, and neurophysiological imaging studies of depression, 135–138

Response conflicts, and ACC function during executive control, 30, 32, 33

Rewards, and fMRI studies of neural circuits in children, 53, 62–63, 71–72

Risk factors, and childhood percursors of adult mental disorders, 56

Sample selection, and neurophysiological imaging studies of depression, 135–138

Scale for Assessment of Negative Symptoms, 101

Scaled Subprofile Model (SSM), 107, 110, 113

Schizophrenia
ACC and performance monitoring in, 41–43
cognitive deficits and, 25

development of brain imaging and studies of, 1–3
executive functions and role of DLPFC and ACC in, 36–43, 46
fMRI studies of mental illness and, 5–8, 10–13, 15–17
N-back working memory and fMRI studies of, 4–5, 39, **40,** 43
prefrontal cortex function and, 2–3, 7–8, 9–13, **14,** 17
signs of in children at risk for, 57
Selective serotonin reuptake inhibitors (SSRIs), and major depression, 139
Serotonin and serotonin system, and neurophysiological imaging studies of depression, 136–137, 150, 156, 157, 158
Sertraline, and late-life depression, 112–113
Single-positron emission computer tomography (SPECT). *See also* [99]Tc hexamethyl propyleneamine oxime (HMPAO) SPECT
ACC and performance monitoring in schizophrenia, 41–42
cerebral blood flow in major depressive disorder and, 131
encephalomalacia and, 95
orbital frontal cortex and symptoms of obsessive-compulsive disorder, 44
Social phobia
facial stimuli and, 70–71

fear conditioning and, 68
Somatosensory cortex, and cerebral blood flow in depression, 129
Sporadic-depressive disease, 125
Stable xenon computed tomography, 95
Statistical parametric mapping (SPM), 12–13
Statistical sensitivity, and analysis methods in brain imaging, 131–132
Sternberg Item Recognition Paradigm, 7
Stimulus-correlated motion (SCM), and periodic task design, 5
Strategic functions. *See also* Executive functions
ACC and performance monitoring, 32
cognitive model of, 27–28, 29
frontal cortex and evaluative processes, **34–35**
Stroop task, **34–35**
Structural MRI studies, of pediatric mood and anxiety disorders, 66–67
Subcortical arteriosclerotic encephalopathy. *See* Encephalomalacia
Subgenual PFC, and depression, 139–144
Suicide
NMDA receptors in prefrontal cortex and, 157
serotonin system and, 137
Sulcal prominence, and late-life depression, 98–99

⁹⁹Tc hexamethyl propyleneamine oxime (HMPAO) SPECT, 95, 106. *See also* Single-positron emission computer tomography

Thalamus, and major depression, 152

Top-down control, of executive functions by DLPFC, 32–36

Treatment response, in late-life depression, 89–90, 110–114

Tricyclic antidepressants, and late-life depression, 98. *See also* Antidepressants

Type I and Type II errors, in neuroimaging literature, 135–136

Unidentified bright objects. *See* Encephalomalacia

Unipolar depression. *See also* Major depressive disorder neuroimaging distinctions and, 125, 156 prefrontal cortex and, 104

Val-Val and Val-Met individuals, and genetic studies of schizophrenia, 10

Ventral anterior cingulate gyrus, and depression, 139–144

Ventral prefrontal cortex, and reward-related behavior, 62. *See also* Prefrontal cortex

Ventricular brain ratio (VBR), and late-life depression, 98–102

Ventrolateral PFC (VLPFC), and depression, 148–151

Ventromedial striatum, and depression, 152

Vigilance, and anxiety disorders in children, 64

Volumetric brain structural abnormalities, and late-life depression, 97–105

Voxel-by-voxel image analysis, 131–132, **133**

Washington University, 124

Whole-brain proton magnetic resonance spectroscopy (¹H-MRSI), 11, 13, 16–17

Wisconsin Card Sorting Test, 2, 10, 38

Working memory (WM). *See also* Memory fMRI studies of N-back form in schizophrenia, 4–5, 39, **40** prefrontal cortex function in schizophrenia and, 3, 12–13, **14,** 38, 39

Xenon inhalation method, 38